Cellular and Molecul Mechanisms of Inflammat

Signal Transductio Inflammatory Cells

VOLUME 3

Cellular and Molecular Mechanisms of Inflammation

Signal Transduction in Inflammatory Cells, Part A

Edited by

Charles G. Cochrane
Department of Immunology
Research Institute of Scripps Clinic
La Jolla, California

Michael A. Gimbrone, Jr.
Department of Pathology
Brigham and Women's Hospital
Harvard Medical School
Boston, Massachusetts

Academic Press, Inc.
Harcourt Brace Jovanovich, Publishers
San Diego New York Boston London Sydney Tokyo Toronto

This book is printed on acid-free paper. ∞

Academic Press, Inc.
1250 Sixth Avenue, San Diego, California 92101-4311

United Kingdom Edition published by
Academic Press Limited
24–28 Oval Road, London NW1 7DX

International Standard Serial Number: 1052-5882

International Standard Book Number: 0-12-150403-4

PRINTED IN THE UNITED STATES OF AMERICA
92 93 94 95 96 97 BB 9 8 7 6 5 4 3 2 1

Table of Contents

Preface

This volume of *Cellular and Molecular Mechanisms of Inflammation* focuses on mechanisms of the transduction of signals linking stimulated receptors and cellular function. This volume is an extension of themes begun in the initial volume of this series, "Receptors of Inflammatory Cells: Structure–Function Relationships," in which were presented the structures of the major types of receptors that produce signals to the interior of the cell.

This volume is dedicated to the pathways of signal transduction involved in stimulating functions of inflammatory cells associated with both host defense and the development of inflammatory injury. The subjects presented are limited. The volume is not intended to deal with signal transduction of growth factor receptors, steroid receptors, or a comprehensive approach to the initiation of DNA expression. Rather, the aim of this volume is the compilation and description of molecules involved in the initial phases of the signal transduction process in inflammatory cells. The first chapter is devoted to receptor–ligand interaction, the kinetics of which form the basis of the switch turning on the signal to the cell. This aspect is too often overlooked in analyses of cellular stimulation, and the techniques employed by Dr. Sklar allow penetrating insights into the initial kinetics of the process. Since a great many signals for inflammatory cells derive from receptor molecules bearing serum transmembrane domains and are coupled during stimulation to nucleotide binding (G) proteins, the second chapter is devoted to the latest information on this important group of proteins with emphasis on low-molecular-weight G proteins. The G proteins are coupled to several important enzyme systems, three of which are presented: phospholipase C, phospholipase D, and phosphatidylinositol 3-kinase. This final enzyme links receptors and G proteins with cellular proliferation and transformation as well as modulation of the cytoskeletal system, while the previous two enzymes mediate a whole host of cellular functions as noted in the chapters. Finally, we have selected two additional areas for discussion since they are central to many functions of inflammatory cells, namely, calcium mobilization and phosphatidylinositol turnover.

It must be recognized that certain facets of signal transduction are not included. Future volumes will deal with these subjects. We ask the reader's indulgence in such omissions with the hope that the presentations in this volume will form a core of information on essential molecular interactions that will provide helpful insights into the initial phases of signal transduction. Another deficiency in this volume is the absence of an analysis of the modulation of activated receptors, including receptors, kinases, and associated molecules such as those of the arrestin series. A requested chapter dedicated to this subject failed to surface and the reader is referred to original texts in the literature.

As in our previous volumes, we have carefully selected the contributors to these subject areas and are indebted to the commitment made by the authors in these highly respected laboratories. We have also, as in previous volumes of this series, directed the contributors not to present a comprehensive list of references, since the series, *Cellular and Molecular Mechanisms of Inflammation,* is dedicated to recent developments.

Charles G. Cochrane
Michael A. Gimbrone, Jr.

CHAPTER 1

Real-Time Analysis of Ligand–Receptor Dynamics and Binding Pocket Structure of the Formyl Peptide Receptor

Larry A. Sklar

Cancer Center, Cytometry
University of New Mexico School of Medicine
Albuquerque, New Mexico 87131 and
Los Alamos National Laboratory

Introduction

We have developed complementary spectrofluorometric and flow cytometric techniques to examine the interactions of formyl peptide ligands (L) with their cell surface receptors (R). These general approaches have now evolved to the point that mechanistic studies based on kinetics of ligand binding and structural insight based on spectroscopic properties of probes

Cellular and Molecular Mechanisms of Inflammation, Volume 3

in binding pockets may now be accessible to the scientific community. These techniques have been used to study ligand–receptor and receptor-processing events in intact neutrophils and ternary complex interactions in permeabilized neutrophils and neutrophil membranes. Kinetic studies suggest that L binds to R at a diffusion-limited rate and that R undergoes rapid transitions involving three states [LR, LRG (the ternary complex of L and R with the G protein), and a desensitized receptor "LRX," which forms within seconds] prior to internalization. A model describing the kinetics of the activation events and based on the real-time methods suggests novel implications in signal transduction via ternary complex pathways. The methodology has also contributed to an understanding of the relationship between receptor occupancy and cell response, including quantitative insight into the details of amplification of intracellular signaling pathways.

Structural information about receptor binding pockets is also now beginning to emerge. We have learned through a spectroscopic analysis of the interaction between L and R that the binding pocket of R is large enough to contain no more than six amino acids and that a fluorescein-labeled pentapeptide is quenched upon binding to R. The quenching appears to be via a static mechanism involving protonation of the chromophore. An analysis of the primary sequence of the receptor suggests points of contact between L and R. We hypothesize that His-90 (putatively located in the extracellular loop connecting the second and third transmembrane domains) protonates L and quenches the probe.

We believe that a number of technological developments will continue to drive the applications and implications of real-time methods. For example, technology being developed at the National Flow Cytometry Resource at Los Alamos National Laboratory is expected to extend and generalize the analysis of receptor structure and dynamics to low-affinity peptide receptors of living biological systems. This technology is expected to be available to support a broad user community.

Birth of Real-Time Assays for Neutrophil Receptor Dynamics

It is now clear that cell activation involves a sequence of transient macromolecular assemblies, beginning with the binding of stimulatory ligands to cell surface receptors. Whereas receptor activities had classically been identified by physiological means, the introduction of radiolabeled ligands permitted a breakthrough in the ability to identify, characterize, and purify receptors. The early phases of our work to develop real-time spectrofluorometric and flow cytometric approaches to analyze neutrophil receptors had their origins in the late 1970s. These investigations were promoted by several important factors. First, it was beginning to be recognized that hormone receptors exhibited guanine nucleotide sensitivity in ligand binding (1). These observations indicated that ligand binding analysis was likely to play an important role in understanding signal transduction as well as being a tool for identifying the distribution of binding sites on various tissues and purifying the molecules. Second, there was at this time considerable interest in the idea that ligand or receptor internalization played a necessary role in signaling for some receptors (2). Niedel *et al.* (3) had just succeeded in preparing a rhodamine derivative of the newly identified chemoattractant formyl peptide and used fluorescence microscopy to visualize its rapid clustering and internalization. Finally, Zigmond and co-workers (4) had engaged upon the arduous task of attempting to unravel the connection between ligand-binding and cell responses for neutrophils chemotaxing in gradients. Their studies made obvious the need to take into account receptor expression or up-regulation, internalization, and recycling.

Our first attempt to understand the relationship between receptor occupancy and neutrophil response began in 1980. At that time a number of convenient assays were available to measure neutrophil responses continuously and in real time. These included recently introduced methods for detection of superoxide generation by cytochrome reduction and membrane depolarization by membrane potential-sensitive dyes. In an effort to understand how signaling might progress through a chemotactic process, we began to consider how cells would respond to a stimulus administered in a temporal gradient (5). That is, to mimic the temporal aspects of increasing stimulus concentration that a cell would encounter while chemotaxing up a spatial gradient, we delivered formyl peptide to cells in suspension, using an infusion pump to ramp the stimulus concentration. We found that the responses elongated in time, but eventually the rates of stimulus administration were so low that the cells failed to respond at all. Using very approximate arguments concerning the rates of ligand binding based on the studies by Zigmond *et al.* and noting the impact of the infusion on the responses, we suggested that low rates of occupancy were required to initiate responses and that chemotaxis might require as few as 1% of the receptors occupied per minute.

These initial observations prompted us to pursue a course toward understanding the relationship between ligand–receptor dynamics and cell response. A number of challenges immediately presented themselves. First, we were aware of a need to make early time, as well as time-dependent, measurements of binding at low levels of receptor occupancy. It was already clear that neutrophils had the capabilities of varying receptor expression in complicated ways (i.e., changing affinity during receptor desensitization and changing number through expression, internalization, and recycling). Investigators before us had already resorted to complex sampling protocols involving binding at one temperature, changing the temperature for the wash step, and changing again for analysis. We were uncertain about particular aspects of radioligand techniques, including the specificity of binding assays with hydrophobic ligands, the ultimate time resolution accessible with heterogeneous assays requiring wash steps, and the difficulty in performing time-dependent assays. As noted, when a number of processing events could proceed simultaneously, it was necessary to use temperature as a tool in trapping individual steps. The possibility of using fluorescent formyl peptides in real-time assays was strengthened for us by several reports of acetylcholine receptor dynamics with fluorescent ligands (6). Preparations of acetylcholine receptor suspended at micromolar concentration had permitted the analysis of agonists and antagonists with affinities comparable to or tighter than the receptor concentration. Would it be similarly possible to examine neutrophil receptors expressed at 50,000 per cell at cell densities up to 10 million per milliliter? In this case, receptor densities were expected to be no more than 1 n*M*!

Early Methods 1980–1985

The key to any real-time binding assay is the ability to discriminate free and bound ligand. Spectrally sensitive probes change absorbance or emission properties when ligands bind to receptors, resulting in wavelength shifts. Spectroscopic changes are also possible, such as a change in fluorescence depolarization resulting from altered rates of rotational relaxation of the free and bound ligand species, a change in intensity (i.e., quenching or enhancement), or a change in fluorescence lifetime. As we were soon to realize, single-cell detection (suggested by the success of the microscopic studies) also made flow cytometric detection reasonable. Not initially realizing the power of flow cytometry, we explored the feasibility of suspension methods in cuvettes. After synthesizing the fluoresceinated hexapeptide, we confronted two problems immediately: how to detect the signal from the ligand in the presence of overwhelming scatter signals from 10 million cells per milliliter and how to resolve the signals emanating from free and bound ligand molecules. Some years earlier I had uncovered a report by Walter Dandliker and colleagues (7) describing high-affinity antibodies to fluorescein which quenched the emission of fluorescein when fluorescein was bound to the antibody. As my co-workers were immunologists, I wondered whether it would be possible to use antibodies to physically discriminate the free and bound ligand. As luck would have it, Dandliker was in the same institution as I, and he willingly provided both advice and reagents. The advice was that, since the cell-bound ligand had been resolved from free ligand and light scatter through microscopy, there was no doubt that filters and monochromators could resolve scatter and fluorescent signal in the cell suspension. The reagent he had available was a preparation of high-affinity polyclonal antibody to fluorescein derived from hyperimmunized rabbits. The antibody proved essential in getting the work off the ground. It was a short time thereafter that we reported the use of the antibody to fluorescein in quenching the free fluoresceinated ligand in the presence of cell-bound ligand (8). Thus, it was possible to achieve a real-time analysis of ligand binding in cell suspensions with the cells and the receptors present at concentrations comparable to their natural abundance. These studies also used the antibody to interrupt cell stimulation during early phases of ligand binding. This was possible because the antibody bound free ligand rapidly, and the resulting complex bound poorly to the cell surface receptors. The results confirmed initial observations that responses were initiated by low levels of occupancy. Since we observed that individual responses required different levels of occupancy, these results began to sow the seeds for us of the concept of divergent pathways of cell response.

At this time flow cytometry was beginning to be used widely among immunologists, and an instrument was available in my institution for pilot studies of formyl peptide binding. The first experiment was designed to answer two questions: Could binding be detected on a single-cell basis, and what impact did washing the free ligand have on the measurement? Even with the instruments of that era, there was no trouble in detecting binding. To our surprise the cytometric signal was not remarkably different if cells labeled with 1 n*M* fluorescent ligand were washed free of the unbound ligand. Moreover, cells exposed to fluorescent ligand in the presence of excess nonfluorescent ligand remained essentially as dim as cells which had never seen the fluorescent ligand. These observations led to a realization that flow cytometry intrinsically discriminated between ligand which had accumulated on the cell surface from ligand dilute in the surrounding solution. The discrimination made possible continuous analysis of cells accumulating or releasing ligand in association or dissociation experiments. Since standards were not available to quantitate receptor numbers in flow cytometry according to the cell brightness, a calibration method was developed at the same time as these initial cytometric investigations (9). The calibration method was based on the idea that total cell binding would vary in response to ligand depletion as a function of varying the cell density.

The introduction of complementary cytometric and fluorometric methodologies set the stage for a systematic investigation of the relationship of receptor binding, processing, and cell response (10–15). These early studies made contributions in three areas of signal transduction. First, we took advantage of the fact that fluorescein emission intensity is sensitive to pH to probe the role of internalization in cell response (10, 11). The measurement depends on the idea that, within the first 3 minutes of binding, internalized ligands are not acidified in receptosomal compartments and retain their fluorescence. However, these internalized ligands are protected from quenching when the extracellular pH is lowered. In contrast, the extracellular ligands are effectively and instantaneously quenched by the pH change. Thus, by lowering the pH of the medium, it was possible to follow the kinetics of internalization in real time as a function of time following binding. In the neutrophil internalization was detected after about 30 sec of ligand binding to the cell and proceeded with a half-time of about 3 min, apparently at a rate independent of ligand concentration.

Comparing the kinetics of initiation of cell responses and the onset of internalization, it was clear in 1982 that internalization was too slow to be the turn-on signal for cell activation. We could also combine the results of pulse stimulation protocols with internalization analysis. In pulse stimulation ligand is administered, and binding to the receptor is then blocked by adding antibody to fluorescein or receptor antagonists (8, 14). We then compared the rate at which responses stopped to the rate at which ligands were cleared from the cell surface by internalization. It was evident from these investigations that internalization was also too slow to be the turn-off step for cell responses because responses had ceased prior to ligand internalization. From kinetic analysis alone, it was appropriate to conclude that receptor activation and desensitization steps were all occurring at a time prior to clearance of receptors from the cell surface.

It was about 1982 when work from a number of laboratories implicated a pathway in which formyl peptide receptors signaled through G proteins. Two types of experiments were reported: Neutrophil membrane preparations exhibited nucleotide-sensitive ligand binding (16) and ligand-stimulated GTPase activities (17). Late in 1984, pertussis toxin was available to demonstrate G protein activities in the neutrophil (18). At the same time, the real-time kinetic studies were beginning to make their second contribution, by revealing time-dependent heterogeneity in ligand–receptor interactions. On the intact cells rapidly dissociating receptor forms were detected within seconds of receptor occupancy, before internalization (14). These rapidly dissociating forms disappeared within tens of seconds. Because the residual slowly dissociating forms were detected at a time when cell responses to pulse stimulation had ceased, these forms appeared to represent the desensitized receptors. It was not until broken-cell preparations were studied in the real-time assays a few years later that it became evident that these rapidly dissociating forms were likely to be receptors uncoupled from G proteins.

Finally, the third contribution of the real-time methods was in the area of occupancy–response relationships. It now became possible to define the number of receptors required to elicit certain cell responses. While it had been appreciated previously that stimulated oxidant production required much higher doses of chemoattractant than chemotaxis, we were able to define occupancy requirements in a considerably more systematic way. We compared real-time binding curves with response levels that had been obtained by using pulse stimulation to define specific levels of occupancy. We found that occupancy of essentially all of the receptors was required to achieve maximal oxidant output (14). In contrast, actin polymerization (15)—and, more recently phosphatidylinositol triphosphate production, which parallels actin polymerization (19)—were stimulated by less than 1% of the receptors. These results have led to a proposal of differential amplification of response pathways, which is considered in more detail below.

To explore the notion that cell responses were sensitive to the rate of ligand binding, sample delivery methods for ligand infusion during cytometric analysis (13) were developed. In studying cell responses, we observed that cytoskeletal responses were still activated when occupancy rates were well below 1% of the receptors per minute; oxidant responses, on the other hand, began to desensitize when occupancy rates fell below about 10% of the receptors per minute (20). These observations suggested to us that there were branch points in the signaling pathways which make it possible for cells to chemotax at low levels of chemoattractant in the vicinity of host tissue without delivering an inflammatory "punch," saving their optimal response capabilities for sites of developing inflammation or host defense where much higher levels of stimulus were available.

Receptor–G Protein Interactions

The treatment of neutrophils with pertussis toxin impairs cell response due to a disruption of coupling between receptors and G proteins. These observations provided the clearest evidence that the first steps of neutrophil activation require an assembly of ternary complex, an interaction among peptide ligands, receptors, and G proteins. We first examined these interactions using spectrofluorometry in digitonin-permeabilized cells (21) by the antibody detection method. In this permeabilized cell preparation a slowly dissociating complex is detected in the presence of ligand and the absence of guanine nucleotide. When guanine nucleotide is present or the G protein is treated with pertussis toxin, a rapidly dissociating receptor is detected. The sensitivity of the binding to guanine nucleotide and pertussis toxin is generally agreed to define the slowly dissociating receptor as the ternary complex LRG and the rapidly dissociating receptor as the binary complex LR. The dissociation rates differed by about two orders of magnitude, LRG dissociating with a half-time of ~500 sec and LR, with a half-time of ~5 sec.

This permeabilized cell preparation was a key element in our work because the ternary complex events can be isolated from subsequent receptor-processing steps which occur in the intact cell. This system also provided our first opportunity to apply kinetic approaches to gain mechanistic insight into ternary complex interactions. We learned that once the ternary complex is formed, its dissociation into LR is rapid following the administration of saturating nucleotide. We analyzed the kinetics of ternary complex disassembly by varying the concentration of guanine nucleotide and examining the rate of dissociation of the ligand (22). The results suggested that, at saturating nucleotide levels, the binding of GTP[S] and the break-up of the ternary complex occur on a subsecond time frame. A more detailed mechanistic analysis was consistent with the notion that the rate-limiting step in the disassembly of the quaternary complex is the binding of the guanine nucleotide to the ternary complex. While, the break-up of the ternary complex occurred too fast to be measured directly by the antibody technique, the results provided some physiological insight. The observations are consistent with the idea that inside a neutrophil (which contains GTP levels of several hundred micromolar), once ternary complex forms, activation of the G protein occurs within 100 msec.

How fast does the ternary complex LRG form? The fact that cell responses are beginning to be detected in the first seconds after stimulus additions implies there is not a significant delay in the transduction process. However, the use of antibodies to discriminate free and bound ligand limits the time resolution of our kinetic analysis. While the method is performed in real time, it is essentially a heterogeneous assay, because the antibody perturbs the distribution of ligand in the system. Moreover, the method does not permit a continuous analysis of the association kinetics. Therefore, to a first approximation, all of the ligand bound to receptor was always detected in the slowly dissociating LRG form when nucleotide was absent. Thus, it really was not rigorously possible to judge whether ternary complex formed rapidly when ligand was added or whether R and G were precoupled in the absence of ligand. Other cuvette methods also suffer from another difficulty. That is, when working at the very high ligand concentrations needed to observe significant formation of low-affinity LR complexes, most of the ligand is free. When ligand concentrations are high and exceed the receptor concentrations, it is harder to detect bound ligand, and, together, these factors compromise the direct analysis of low-affinity LR interactions.

Recently, we succeeded in analyzing ternary complex interactions by two more effective approaches using kinetic applications of flow cytometry (23) and spectrofluorometry with ligands whose fluorescence is quenched upon binding to the receptor (unpublished observations). Both of these detection systems are rigorously homogeneous, and although the cytometric time resolution is limited to about 5 sec, a detailed kinetic analysis of ligand–receptor interactions has been possible (23). The cytometric method is particularly useful when working at comparatively high ligand concentrations and low-affinity binding interactions, because of the intrinsic ability of the analysis to detect cell-associated ligand and to discriminate free ligand in the bulk environment. This occurs because data acquisition is triggered by the presence of a cell, and the ligand in the volumes between cells is essentially ignored.

Equilibrium binding studies performed by cytometry showed that LRG binds ligand more tightly by two orders of magnitude than LR. A second class of binding sites of smaller number was detected in the absence of guanine nucleotide. The second class of sites has affinity characteristics similar to those of LR, suggesting that some fraction of LR sites remain uncoupled from G in the absence of guanine nucleotide. The presence of receptor sites that do not couple to G protein or couple quite slowly is common to other receptor systems (24) and may actually be rather common. The observation was somewhat surprising for us in view of the fact that, by enzyme-linked immunosorbent assay, there is a 100-fold excess of what appear to be the appropriate G proteins as compared to the receptors (25, 26).

Kinetic studies performed by cytometry (23) have revealed that this change in affinity was due principally to an increase in the dissociation rate constants for LRG (1×10^{-3} sec^{-1}) as compared to LR (1×10^{-1} sec^{-1}). In contrast, the association rate constants for LRG and LR (~3×10^{7} M^{-1} sec^{-1}) were statistically indistinguishable and close to the diffusion limit. Kinetic data have now been fit with a number of models related to the ternary complex. When fit with the simplest one-step reversible binding models, there were systematic errors in the fits, and the predicted off-rate differed by an order of magnitude from the direct measurement of the dissociation of LRG. Only when a full ternary complex model is used do the data systematically fit. The results of the ternary complex analysis, performed on a Cray supercomputer (Mendota Heights, MN), are consistent with a reaction mechanism for the assembly of the LRG ternary complex in which a large fraction of G (about 50%) is precoupled to R and a comparable fraction of R associates slowly (with a half-time of approximately minutes) to form LRG. A similar conclusion was obtained from spectrofluorometric analysis (unpublished observations).

The suggestion of precoupled RG sites is a theoretical possibility implicit in ternary complex analysis, even though solubilized receptors and G proteins do not coisolate on gradients unless ligand is present. Whether there is coupling between R and G on cell surfaces in the absence of ligand has yet to be demonstrated unequivocally to our knowledge. The existence of precoupled RG sites offers the possibility of rapid signal transduction without the need for intervening diffusion of the transduction partners prior to activation. The slowly coupling or uncoupled receptors would appear to reflect a population of receptor sites which are relatively isolated from the transduction pathway. There are two interesting implications of these possibilities. First, there is considerable interest in drug molecules that interfere with RG coupling to be used to control cell response. The utility of such molecules would clearly by limited under conditions in which there are precoupled RG complexes. Second, temporal heterogeneity in cell response might arise as a consequence of there being both precoupled and slowly coupling receptor populations. This is an interesting issue for neutrophils in which some responses are temporally biphasic, the most notable being receptor-stimulated actin polymerization (15, 19). Early actin responses may arise from ligand binding to precoupled RG complexes and late responses from ligand binding to slowly coupling receptors.

We are now engaged in the analysis of ternary complex formation under several types of conditions. Preliminary analysis of the results when guanine nucleotide is at concentrations below saturation of the G proteins suggests that, in the absence of ligand, GTP[S] may mediate a redistribution of the sites defined as uncoupled R and precoupled RG. Although this analysis is as yet incomplete, it provides some tantalizing possibilities.

The calculations that suggest a potential ability of GTP[S] to alter the coupling between precoupled RG complexes in the absence of ligand have their own implications. They provide a possibility that, in the intact cell, a stable resting form of R and G exists without nucleotide "RG^-" and that ligand causes the empty G site to open to accommodate the nucleotide. I have always wondered how it is that GTP[S] can activate responses in broken-cell preparations if ligand is required to catalyze the release of endogenous GDP, which is often thought to be prebound to G proteins. Is there an alternative possibility, that there is some fraction of empty G proteins which are already receptor bound and that GTP[S] is capable of occupying the empty site and activating the G protein without the need for ligand?

Intact Cell

Measurements of receptor dynamics in the intact cell are considerably more complex than in the permeabilized cell because of receptor processing of several kinds. In the neutrophil this includes up-regulation of receptors from secretory granule stores, desensitization of membrane-bound receptors, and internalization of desensitized receptors. We have recently evaluated the up-regulation of receptors in neutrophils in several types of physiologically relevant settings. In blood the receptors in the cells exist primarily in internal storage locations, where they can be up-regulated rapidly by massive degranulation (30,000 per minute), slowly by priming agents such as lipopolysaccharide (halftime of ~ 15 min), or during cell stimulation over 2–3 min (10,000 per minute) by formyl peptides themselves (27). To avoid the complication of the contribution of up-regulation during our measurements, we examined cell preparations in which exposure to optimal lipopolysaccharide concentration during cell isolation from blood leads to expression of the receptors.

In the intact cell the identification of individual receptor states is complicated by spontaneous transduction and processing events. While there has been an increasing understanding of the processing of individual members of the family of G-linked receptors (28), at the time during which we began to characterize receptor states in the cell, the sequence of the formyl peptide receptor had not yet been established. Many of us in this field believed that it would turn out to be a member of the family of receptors which interacted with G proteins possessing seven transmembrane α-helical domains. In several receptors of this type, desensitization involves phosphorylation of serine and threonine residues through specific receptor kinases.

Based on functional measurements defining a slowly dissociating desensitized receptor (LRX) and broken-cell measurements defining uncoupled and G-coupled forms, there are compelling arguments for three different receptor forms in the intact cell (29). To identify these forms in the cell, we undertook a strategy to trap the distinct receptor forms. We believed that RG interactions would be sensitive to pertussis toxin, while desensitized receptor forms dependent on receptor phosphorylation would be sensitive to cellular energy levels. The measurements of ligand–receptor interaction for such studies only required an analysis of ligand off-rates in response to treatment of the cells by pertussis toxin and metabolic inhibitors. Thus, we could take advantage of the antibody technology. The results (Fig. 1) of these experiments suggested that the slowly dissociating receptor form detected in the intact cell after activation, but prior to internalization (i.e., the desensitized receptor), was, in fact, the major receptor form detected at 37°C. We found that, while the formation of the desensitized form requires energy, direct evidence of phosphorylation of the formyl peptide receptor had not yet been obtained. When cellular energy levels are depleted, and adenine and guanine nucleotide levels fall, LRG can be formed. This occurs presumably because the lack of ATP inhibits desensitization of the receptors, and the lack of free guanine nucleotide permits stabilization of LRG. The identity of the second slowly dissociating receptor form distinct from LRX as LRG is confirmed by the idea that low energy levels block LRX formation and ribosylation blocks LRG formation. In this case a rapidly dissociating receptor with the characteristics previously ascribed to LR is detected. Moreover, experiments

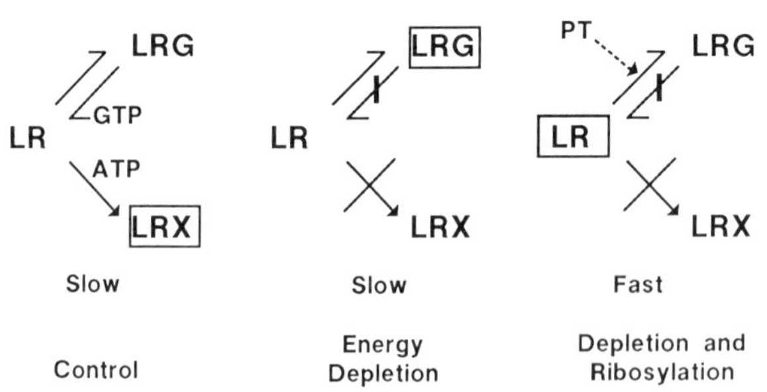

FIGURE 1

Three receptor forms have been identified: a slowly dissociating desensitized LRX, a rapidly dissociating LR, and the slowly dissociating LRG. In the cell the interconversions from LRG and LR are mediated by guanine nucleotide; the formation of LRX depends on energy (probably through ATP-dependent phosphorylation). Under normal circumstances LRX forms spontaneously and dominates the observed ligand–receptor interactions. By poisoning energy metabolism, LRG is trapped, because levels of both adenine and guanine nucleotides fall. Through the combination of pertussis toxin (PT) treatment (uncoupling receptors from G proteins) and energy depletion, LR is formed.

with ribosylation by pertussis toxin indicate that, while occupancy by agonist is required for receptor desensitization, neither G protein nor cell activation is required to form LRX.

Because of the considerable interest in the role of the cytoskeleton in regulating ligand–receptor interaction, we examined cells treated with *Clostridium botulinum* C_2 toxin. This toxin blocks receptor-stimulated actin polymerization and reduces resting levels of F-actin to virtually undetectable levels. Since the desensitized receptor state forms more or less normally in cells depleted of F-actin by treatment with *C. botulinum* C_2 toxin (30), it appears that microfilaments are not absolutely required for desensitization.

Given the information now available concerning the behavior of ternary complex in permeabilized cells, and the identification of distinct receptor forms in intact cells and their regulation, it is appropriate to develop a whole-cell model of ligand–receptor interactions. To analyze and model ligand–receptor interactions in intact cells, several additional technical demands must be satisfied. First, in the intact cells it is necessary to take into account the fact that interconversions among all three receptor forms occur rapidly. Analysis of these interconversions requires technology which permits continuous analysis of ligand association and dissociation in the 1-sec time frame. As indicated, the antibody technique is better suited to the dissociation process; however, the time resolution in flow cytometry with existing instrumentation is not entirely adequate for the needs of second or subsecond time resolution. Second, ligand–receptor complexes are internalized. Assay systems that permit continuous analysis of ligand association and dissociation use fluorescence polarization on cells suspended in cuvettes (31, 32) or take advantage of probes that change intensity upon binding to the receptor (33). The internalization assay takes advantage of fluorescein as a pH indicator and uses a rapid pH change as a quench step to identify extracellular ligand (11, 12).

In contrast to the broken-cell system, in the intact cell there is a rapid spontaneous interconversion among the three receptor states, with rapid formation of the desensitized receptor LRX (29). The evolution among the receptor states can be probed in the following manner. After the fluorescent ligand is added to the cell suspension, a nonfluorescent antagonist follows at distinct times after the fluorescent agonist. At early times in the ligand binding, a rapidly dissociating form similar to LR is followed by a slowly dissociating desensitized receptor, LRX. After 1 min or so of binding to the receptor, only the slowly dissociating receptor is detected. Direct measurements of internalization indicate that the slowly dissociating receptor is internalized somewhat more slowly, with a half-time of 3 min following a delay of about 30 sec.

The observed data can be fit with a model based on the direct observation of the behavior of LR and LRG in the permeabilized cell combined with the behavior of LRX and internalization in the intact cell [Eq. (1)]. From the permeabilized cell we learn that ligand finds receptor at a rate of $3 \times 10^7\ M^{-1}\ \text{sec}^{-1}$. Receptors exist in forms which rapidly couple to G (or are precoupled) and those which are uncoupled from G (and may slowly couple). At concentrations of guanine nucleotide expected to be present inside the cell, activation via transient formation of the LRG•GTP quaternary complex is expected at a rate of more than 10 per second. From the intact cell we learn that the uncoupled receptor desensitizes (LRX) at a rate estimated to be 0.1 per second. LRX is slowly dissociating and is subsequently internalized with ligand associated.

The analysis is consistent with these concepts: (1) The LRG which contributes to early signals disappears within 1 sec during cell activation in the intact cell, which is too rapid for LRG to be detected with the time resolution available; (2) the dynamics observed in the intact cell appear to be dominated by a rapid interconversion between the rapidly dissociating LR and the slowly dissociating LRX. The interconversion occurs in several seconds. But where is LR coming from? LR could arise as the product of ternary complex which has been activated and then disassembles, or LR could arise as a consequence of ligand binding to receptors which couple slowly to G proteins. The extent of cell activation would then depend both on the fraction of receptors partitioned between forms which are precoupled to G and uncoupled from G and on the relative rate at which receptors which are uncoupled from G either couple or become desensitized.

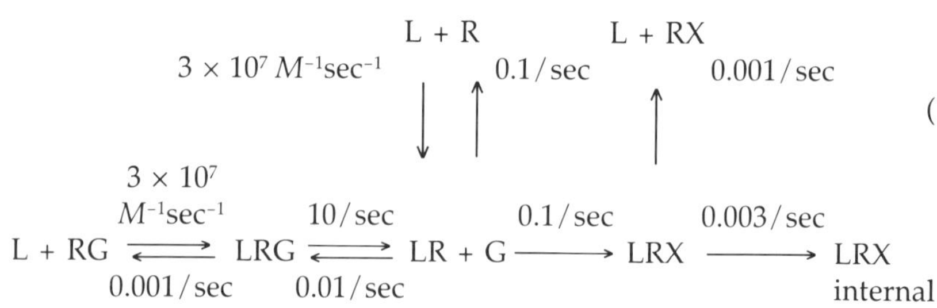

(1)

Calculations based on the behavior of the ternary complex [Eq. (1)] in the intact cell have been performed. During ligand binding the total amount of active LRG rises rapidly to a maximum within tens of seconds, then decays slowly over several minutes as binding approaches "equilibrium." (It is difficult to think of the binding in the intact cell as strictly an equilibrium, since there appear to be two largely irreversible steps: desensitization and internalization.) When binding of an agonist is interrupted by applying a saturating concentration of an antagonist (or adding the antibody to fluorescein), the calculations show that the ternary complex decays rapidly, within seconds (31, 32). Under normal conditions cell stimulation is accompanied by cell responses which are initiated within a few seconds, reach maximal rates of response within tens of seconds, then decay slowly over periods of minutes (14). When agonist binding is interrupted, it takes a few seconds for the response to be affected, then the response decays. We believe that the cell responses decay because the transduction pathway collapses once the active forms of the receptor have been lost. Thus, it appears that the behavior of the active receptor forms is relatively consistent with cell response behavior.

Taken together, it appears that LR dynamics can be accounted for in a semiquantitative manner by combining the ternary complex behavior observed in the permeabilized cell with identification of the receptor states in the intact cell. At the present time, however, an important piece of the puzzle is missing: the description of the extent to which receptors are either coupled to or uncoupled from G proteins in the intact cell during stimulation. In Eq. (1) the coexistence of uncoupled R and precoupled RG would be reflected by the fraction of ligands entering the activation pathway to form either LR or LRG. Since the disappearance of LRG is fast for the entry in the RG arm, the receptor dynamics appear to be dominated by the interconversions between LR and LRX. As long as LRG disappears rapidly, the mathematical characteristics of the entry into the pathway as LR or LRG are identical with respect to R. Entry via the LRG arms leads to efficient activation, while entry in the LR arm leads to inefficient activation. Experimentally, we are as yet unable to resolve the issue of heterogeneity of RG coupling in the intact cell on the basis of ligand binding dynamics. On the other hand, biochemical evidence (discussed below) suggests that formyl peptide receptors do not appear to activate a large number of G proteins sequentially (26). This observation is consistent with the idea that uncoupled receptors, whether they have become uncoupled after ternary complex activation or have yet to find a G protein, are more likely to be desensitized than to find a G protein to produce another round of activation signals.

Amplification

We have tried to integrate the results available from the real-time binding methodology with pulse stimulation to generate concepts of amplification in the stimulatory neutrophil pathways (14, 15, 19, 26, 34). These studies led to the notion that there was remarkable amplification in the stimulatory pathways, with a single receptor leading simultaneously to the polymerization of an estimated 100,000 actins and the production of 100,000 radicals of superoxide (34). While superficially similar on a quantitative basis, amplification in these pathways depends on profoundly different molecular details. Each pathway appears to show a common dependence on the pertussis toxin-sensitive G proteins required for signal transduction. Amplification at the level of G protein activation appears to be minimal. Each formyl peptide receptor with access to G proteins appears to stimulate the hydrolysis of a small number of GTPs per minute (26). This notion of limited amplification is consistent with the results of ligand–receptor dynamics, in which it appears that receptors are desensitized with a half-time of ~10 sec and that receptors uncoupled from G proteins may find G proteins only over a period of minutes. We hypothesize that, once uncoupled, formyl peptide receptors are more likely to be desensitized than to find a G protein to initiate a signal cascade. Amplification in the oxidant pathway is projected (34) to arise from the ability of an activated G protein to activate a single phospholipase C long enough to produce hundreds to thousands of hydrolyzed phosphatidylinositols. A cascade generating thousands of soluble inositol phosphates and diacylglycerols releases tens of thousands of free calcium ions, activates large numbers of protein kinase C, and ultimately assembles sufficient oxidase complexes for the oxidant burst. There is enough signaling capacity in the pathway to respond to occupancy of virtually all of the expressed receptors.

In contrast, after ~100 receptors have been occupied, 10 million actins become polymerized, representing the net capacity of the cell. The actin pathway appears to be independent of intracellular calcium and may reflect an independent signaling branch in which G proteins activate, either directly or indirectly, a phosphatidylinositol 3-kinase pathway (19). The actin pathway is remarkably biphasic with respect to receptor occupancy and time course of response. Beyond the first hundred receptors it is the duration of the response which elongates, rather than its magnitude. It is conceivable that the second phase of response represents the fraction of receptors which only couple to G slowly and relatively inefficiently as they are partitioned into the desensitized receptor pool. Such a hypothesis implies that differences in time courses of actin polymerization for different chemoattractant receptor types could be related to heterogeneity in access to the G proteins.

Neutrophils also possess an inhibitory pathway which blunts the oxidant output of the stimulatory pathway, without significant impact on the actin pathway. The output of 500 β-adrenergic receptors compromises the output of 50,000 formyl peptide receptors (35). How do 500 receptors block 50,000? GTPase analysis suggests that occupying the adrenergic receptors leads to a comparable net GTPase activity as the formyl peptide receptors (26). Since the adrenergic receptors are expressed at only 1% of the level of formyl peptide receptors, the amplification may be 100 times greater through the β-adrenergic receptor as compared to the formyl peptide receptor. We propose that there may be an activation of 100 G_s's for each adrenergic receptor as compared to one G_i for each formyl peptide receptor. The inhibitory pathway proceeds through production of an estimated 10,000 cAMPs for each activated receptor (26). The number of A kinases activated is as yet unknown, but a potential target of the A kinase is a RAP protein, which may be a regulatory subunit of the oxidase itself (36). Thus, as a working hypothesis, we suggest that a highly amplified inhibitory pathway intersects a stimulatory pathway at a common regulatory site.

Ligand–Receptor Dynamics for Unlabeled Ligands

There are a number of circumstances in which labeled ligands are not available for studies of ligand–receptor interactions. In some cases ligands are available, but the measurements are difficult because the binding affinities are too low. For these reasons we developed a cytometric approach to extract rate constants for nonlabeled ligands. The concept of the method is that, since binding affinities for unlabeled ligands can be determined from equilibrium analysis of competition between labeled and unlabeled molecules, then the kinetic aspects of the competition can be used to evaluate the rate constants for the unlabeled ligands. A series of nonfluorescent peptide agonists and antagonists was studied in competition with a fluorescent agonist (37). We concluded that the antagonists were characterized by subsecond residence times at the receptor, while the agonists have long and time-dependent residence times. In light of more detailed information, we would now interpret the time-dependent loss of dissociability of agonists as reflecting the receptor-processing events of signal transduction, including formation of the desensitized receptor.

An approach based on the functional capabilities of the antagonists was used to estimate the association rates of antagonists with the formyl peptide receptor (37). These experiments depend on an analysis of the rate at which cell response to agonists was inhibited by antagonists. The results yielded conclusions about antagonist binding rate constants similar to those derived from the competitive binding studies. This approach was subsequently extended to the analysis of ligands which initiated the inhibitory pathway (35). Rate constants for the binding and dissociation of the β-adrenergic receptors were estimated from the rates at which the catecholamines inhibited the function of formyl peptide receptors. To our knowledge the calculated rates represented the first estimate for the binding of isoproterenol to cells at physiological temperature. The results suggested that agonists for both stimulatory and inhibitory receptors interact with their specific receptors at rates approaching the diffusion limit.

Receptor Binding Pocket Topography

The development of experimental conditions for detecting ligand–receptor interactions by fluorescence methods provides the possibility for making spectroscopic measurements from probes within the binding pockets of receptors. Spectroscopy can be a link to molecular structure, because the fluorescence properties of probes are sensitive to the molecular environment of the site. We have begun to take advantage of these capabilities to study the topography of interaction of a family of fluorescent formyl peptides containing four (CHO–Met–Leu–Phe–Lys–fluorescein), five (CHO–Met–Leu–Phe–Phe–Lys–fluorescein), and six (CHO–Nle–Leu–Phe–Nle–Tyr–Lys–fluorescein and CHO–Met–Leu–Phe–Phe–Phe–Lys–fluorescein) amino acids with their receptor, using spectroscopic methods (33). The fluorescent peptides containing four and five amino acids were quenched upon binding to the receptor, indicating interaction of the chromophore with the receptor. In contrast, the hexapeptides were accessible to antibodies to fluorescein. Taken together, these results suggest that the C terminus of the tetrapeptide or the pentapeptide is protected in the receptor binding pocket, while the fluorescein on the C terminus of either hexapeptide is exposed and recognized by the antibody to fluorescein. These results indicate that the binding pocket accommodates at least five but no more than six amino acids.

To understand the structural basis of the quenching interaction in the receptor binding pocket, we have investigated the spectroscopy of the bound fluorescein. We examined the fluorescence lifetime of the fluoresceinated ligand probes in and out of the binding pocket. The measurements provide insight into whether the quenching occurred by a static or dynamic mechanism and the structure of the binding pocket responsible for the quenching. In dynamic quenching the fluorescence lifetime and quantum yield would vary in parallel and would suggest that the environment of the fluorescein in the binding pocket was fluctuating on the time frame of the fluorescein lifetime (~4 nsec). In the binding pocket, however, we detected residual long lifetime for the pentapeptide, rather than intermediate fluorescent lifetime (unpublished observations). This result suggests a static quenching mechanism in which the probe exists in either a quenched (short lifetime) or unquenched (long native lifetime) state. Two molecular mechanisms can account for coexisting environments: Fluorescein can be quenched by a hydrophobic pocket, in which case static quenching could require some probe molecules in the pocket and some outside; or fluorescein can be quenched by protonation, in which case coexisting protonated and unprotonated forms would be detected. It is expected that fluorescein in a hydrophobic pocket will exhibit a blue-shifted emission spectrum. In preliminary measurements no shift of the emission spectrum was detected, consistent with protonatin mechanism. We have also now examined the pH dependence of the fluorescence of the bound peptide (38). The tetrapeptide was unresponsive to pH, while the pentapeptide was quenched with a pKa of ~7.5, consistent with interaction with an interfacial histidine residue.

The formyl peptide receptor has been recently cloned and sequenced (39). The receptor appears to possess seven transmembrane α-helical domains, like the β-adrenergic receptor and the photoreceptor rhodopsin. In these receptors the binding pocket is located in a cleft about one-third of the way across the membrane bilayer formed by the α-helical domains. The expected peptide binding region is rich in aromatic amino acids, and there is a single histidine (His-90) located in a short loop connecting the second and third transmembrane domains, perhaps 10–15 Å from the aromatic acid-rich binding pocket. His-90 is a good candidate for a proton donor responsible for quenching the fluorescein of the pentapeptide, while the tetrapeptide may be quenched by interactions with nearby aromatic amino acids. We are presently engaged in producing probe molecules that will exhibit distinct characteristics in hydrophobic, as compared to protonating, environments. It might ultimately be possible to engage chromophores in conformationally active domains of the binding pocket of the receptors, leading to detection of the intramolecular transitions required for signal transduction.

Prospects for Generalizing Real-Time Methods for Kinetic and Structural Analyses

In the previous sections I suggested that fluorescence methodology offers the promise of analyzing ligand–receptor interactions in living systems at the natural abundance of cell surface receptors. The example discussed, the formyl peptide receptor, can bind agonists with affinities up to $10^{10}\ M^{-1}$, and 50,000 or more receptors are expressed on a fully activated neutrophil. From a technological perspective it would be desirable to extend the methodology to ligands with affinities as low as $10^6\ M^{-1}$. This range of affinities would encompass most hormone systems and the binding of synthetic peptides and peptidomimetics. Flow cytometric methods are intrinsically suited to these goals, since, in flowing systems, data acquisition is triggered by the presence of a cell or particle and its accompanying light-scatter signal. Thus, flow cytometry is uniquely suited to discriminating the signals of fluorescent ligands associated with cells from the signal of the fluorescent ligands in dilute solution surrounding the cells. Nonetheless, there are limits to the detection of bound ligands: (1) when a small number of ligands are bound per cell or when the ligand fluorescence associated with the cells is not significantly more intense than the cell autofluorescence; or (2) when the binding affinity of the ligand is low, so that a high ligand concentration is required to saturate the binding sites.

Using commercial cytometers and cell preparations which are not highly autofluorescent (e.g., blood cells, but not tissue culture cells) the binding of 10,000 fluorescein-labeled ligands can be detected if the affinity is $10^8\ M^{-1}$ or higher. However, if the affinity is $10^6\ M^{-1}$, 1 million sites must be present. In general, the higher the affinity of the ligand binding, the lower the number of sites required for detection. There is, however, a variety of approaches to improving the sensitivity of detection. For example, chemistry allows the development of probes with emission properties distinct from cell autofluorescence. Instrumental developments provide computational, electronic, and optical approaches to extending these limits. For instance, instrumentation at the National Flow Cytometry Resource is being developed to discriminate chromophores on the basis of their spectrum (wavelength) (40) or fluorescence lifetime.

A more general approach involves cytometers with fast-mixing capabilities. For small molecules of affinity $10^6\ M^{-1}$, typical association and dissociation rates are predicted to be $\leq 10^7\ M^{-1}\text{sec}^{-1}$ and $\leq 10\ \text{sec}^{-1}$. For such low-affinity molecules the equilibration times are governed by the dissociation rates, which, in general, will be in the time frame (i.e., half-time) of ~100 msec. Flow cytometric detection systems, particularly with the new digital data acquisition systems being built at the National Flow Cytometry Resource, can be equipped to function on this time frame. The most serious limitations presently arise from sample mixing and delivery times, which generally require several seconds. With high-affinity ligands and substantial receptor numbers it will be possible, with fast mixing, to directly examine kinetics of binding and macromolecular assembly. In the case of low-affinity ligands with low receptor number, one could imagine premixing the cells with ligand, then rapidly diluting the cells prior to the cytometric analysis. The dilution would wash away the concentrated ligand, and the analysis of ligand spectroscopy and kinetic ligand–receptor processes could be performed during the course of ligand dissociation from its receptor. Fast-mixing technology has existed for more than 50 years in the physico-chemical literature. The next generation of cytometers should be able to incorporate analysis in the tens to hundreds of milliseconds by adding stopped-flow or continuous-flow injection capabilities. In fact, a recent demonstration of microsecond mixing in cell-sized volumes (41) suggests that it may ultimately become possible to visualize protein conformation dynamics in cell–receptor systems in the microsecond time domain. In this time domain we expect to examine binding mechanisms and receptor structural reorganization associated with binding events.

On a more immediate level it will also be possible to apply fast-mixing technology directly to macromolecular assemblies. For systems in which it is already possible to resolve free and bound ligand, such as the formyl peptide receptor, using ligand molecules that are quenched upon binding to the receptor, it should shortly be possible to examine a variety of subsecond nucleotide-dependent events. These include analysis of the formation of LR and analysis of the lifetime of the quaternary complex following the association of nucleotide with ternary complex. Issues such as the discrimination of precoupled and uncoupled receptors and the activation of G proteins by dissociation into subunits are likely to require not only rapid mixing, but probes for both the R and G transduction partners.

Acknowledgments

I would like to thank Shawn P. Fay and Richard G. Posner for helpful discussions. This work was supported by National Institutes of Health grants AI 19032 and RR 01315.

References

1. A. De Lean, J. M. Stadel, and R. J. Lefkowitz, *J. Biol. Chem.* **255,** 7108–7117 (1980).
2. M. Das and C. F. Fox, *Proc. Natl. Acad. Sci. U.S.A.* **75,** 2644–2648 (1978).
3. J. E. Niedel, S. Wilkinson, and P. Cuatrecasas, *J. Biol. Chem.* **254,** 10700–10706 (1979).
4. S. H. Zigmond, *J. Cell Biol.* **88,** 644–647 (1981).

5. L. A. Sklar, A. J. Jesaitis, R. G. Painter, and C. G. Cochrane, *J. Biol. Chem.* **256,** 9909–9914 (1981).
6. T. Heidmann and J.-P. Changeux, *J. Biochem. (Tokyo)* **94,** 255–279 (1979).
7. S. A. Levison, A. N. Hicks, A. J. Portmann, and W. B. Dandliker, *Biochemistry* **14,** 3778–3786 (1975).
8. L. A. Sklar, Z. G. Oades, A. J. Jesaitis, R. G. Painter, and C. G. Cochrane, *Proc. Natl. Acad. Sci. U.S.A.* **78,** 7540–7544 (1981).
9. L. A. Sklar and D. Finney, *Cytometry* **3,** 161–165 (1982).
10. L. A. Sklar, A. J. Jesaitis, R. G. Painter, and C. G. Cochrane, *J. Cell. Biochem.* **20,** 193–202 (1982).
11. D. A. Finney and L. A. Sklar, *Cytometry* **4,** 54–60 (1983).
12. L. A. Sklar, D. A. Finney, Z. G. Oades, A. J. Jesaitis, R. G. Painter, and C. G. Cochrane, *J. Biol. Chem.* **259,** 5661–5669 (1984).
13. G. M. Omann, W. Coppersmith, D. A. Finney, and L. A. Sklar, *Cytometry* **6,** 69–73 (1985).
14. L. A. Sklar, P. A. Hyslop, Z. G. Oades, G. Omann, A. J. Jesaitis, R. G. Painter, and C. G. Cochrane, *J. Biol. Chem.* **260,** 11461–11467 (1985).
15. L. A. Sklar, G. M. Omann, and R. G. Painter, *J. Cell Biol.* **101,** 1161–1166 (1985).
16. C. Koo, R. J. Lefkowitz, and R. Snyderman, *Biochem. Biophys. Res. Commun.* **106,** 224–229 (1982).
17. P. A. Hyslop, Z. G. Oades, A. J. Jesaitis, R. G. Painter, C. G. Cochrane, and L. A. Sklar, *FEBS Lett.* **166,** 165–169 (1984).
18. G. M. Bokoch and A. G. Gilman, *Cell* **39,** 301–308 (1984).
19. M. Eberle, A. E. Traynor-Kaplan, L. A. Sklar, and J. Norgauer, *J. Biol. Chem.* **265,** 16725–16728 (1990).
20. G. M. Omann and L. A. Sklar, *J. Cell Biol.* **107,** 951–958 (1988).
21. L. A. Sklar, G. M. Bokoch, D. Button, and J. E. Smolen, *J. Biol. Chem.* **262,** 135–139 (1987).
22. L. A. Sklar, W. N. Swann, S. P. Fay, and Z. G. Oades, *in* "Biology of Cellular Transducing Signals," (J. Y. Vanderhoek, ed.) pp. 1–10. Plenum, New York, 1990.
23. S. P. Fay, R. G. Posner, W. N. Swann, and L. A. Sklar, *Biochemistry* **30,** 5066–5075 (1991).
24. R. R. Neubig, R. D. Gantzos, and W. J. Thomsen, *Biochemistry* **27,** 2374–2384 (1988).
25. R. Weingarten, L. Ransnas, L. A. Sklar, and G. M. Bokoch, *J. Biol. Chem.* **265,** 11044–11048 (1990).
26. H. Mueller, R. Weingarten, L. Ransnas, G. M. Bokoch, and L. A. Sklar, *J. Biol. Chem.* **266,** 12939–12943 (1991).
27. J. Norgauer, M. Eberle, S. P. Fay, H.-D. Lemke, and L. A. Sklar, *J. Immunol.* **146,** 975–980 (1991).
28. C. D. Strader, I. S. Sigal, and R. A. F. Dixon, *FASEB J.* **3,** 1825–1832 (1989).
29. L. A. Sklar, H. Mueller, G. M. Omann, and Z. G. Oades, *J. Biol. Chem.* **264,** 8483–8386 (1989).
30. J. Norgauer, K. Aktories, and L. A. Sklar, *J. Cell Biol.* **109,** 1133–1140 (1989).
31. L. A. Sklar, *Annu. Rev. Biophys. Biophys. Chem.* **16,** 479–506 (1987).
32. L. A. Sklar, H. Mueller, W. N. Swann, C. H. Comstock, G. M. Omann, and G. M. Bokoch, *ACS Symp. Ser.* **383,** 52–69 (1989).
33. L. A. Sklar, S. P. Fay, B. E. Seligmann, R. J. Freer, and H. M. Mueller, *Biochemistry* **2,** 313–316 (1990).
34. L. A. Sklar, *Adv. Immunol.* **39,** 95–143 (1986).
35. H. Mueller, H. J. Motulsky, and L. A. Sklar, *Mol. Pharmacol.* **34,** 347–353 (1988).
36. L. A. Quilliam, H. Mueller, B. P. Bohl, V. Prossnitz, L. A. Sklar, C. J. Der, G. M. Bokoch, *J. Immunol.* **147,** 1628–1635 (1991).

37. L. A. Sklar, J. Sayre, V. M. McNeil, and D. A. Finney, *Mol. Pharmacol.* **28,** 323–330 (1985).
38. S. P. Fay, M. Domalewski, D. Magde, R. J. Freer, T. Yoshida, T. Buican, and L. A. Sklar, *Abstr. Congr. Int. Soc. Anal. Cytol., 15th* Suppl. **5,** 60 (1991).
39. F. Boulay, M. Tardif, L. Brouchon, and P. Vignais, *Biochem. Biophys. Res. Commun.* **168,** 1103–1109 (1990).
40. T. N. Buican, *in* "Clinical Cytometry and Histometry" (G. Burger and J. S. Ploem, eds.), pp. 67–71. Academic Press, Orlando, Florida, 1987.
41. P. Regenfuss, R. M. Clegg, M. J. Fulwyler, F. J. Barrantes, and T. M. Jovin, *Rev. Sci. Instrum.* **56,** 283–290 (1985).

CHAPTER 2

Structure and Function of GTP-Binding Proteins in Neutrophil Signal Transduction

Lawrence A. Quilliam and Gary M. Bokoch

Departments of Immunology and Cell Biology
Research Institute of Scripps Clinic
La Jolla, California 92037

Introduction

Neutrophils (polymorphonuclear leukocytes) and macrophages play a major role in the body's defense against harmful foreign pathogens. In the course of serving this function, phagocytes must respond to a variety of inflammatory stimulants, including N-formylated peptides, complement component C5a, leukotriene B_4, platelet-activating factor, and interleukin 8 (1). Phagocytes have specific cell surface receptors for these factors that are coupled to the intracellular environment through oligomeric GTP-binding (G) proteins. These transducing elements are found in all cells and couple ligand-activated receptors to the intracellular second messenger cascades (2). Protein purification and molecular cloning have revealed the existence of multiple additional G proteins that bear homology with the *ras* oncogene products (3, 4). These smaller monomeric proteins are referred to herein as low-molecular-weight G proteins (LMWGs). Recent findings have implicated the LMWGs in a variety of neutrophil activities.

The biochemistry of oligomeric G proteins has recently been the topic of several excellent reviews (2, 5–7), and their role in signal transduction is well characterized. Therefore, in this chapter we put more emphasis on the properties of the LMWGs whose roles in neutrophil function are currently being investigated.

Oligomeric G Proteins

Structure–Function Relationship

The signal-transducing G proteins are heterotrimers that consist of α, β, and γ subunits. Gα's range in size from 39 to 52 kDa, bind guanine nucleotides, and possess an intrinsic GTPase activity. These α subunits have been attributed with both the specificity of receptor recognition and the activation of effector enzymes or ion channels (2, 5).

Studies with α subunit proteins have defined a region near the C terminus to be important for the recognition of both receptors and effectors. Pertussis toxin-catalyzed ADP ribosylation of a cysteine four residues from the C terminus prevents receptor–$G\alpha_i$ protein coupling (see Ref. 2). Further, a mutant form of $G\alpha_S$ that is found in the *unc* variant of S49 lymphoma cells, which do not respond to β-adrenergic receptor activation, has a point mutation close to its C terminus (residue 372) (8). Antibodies raised to C-terminal peptides of Gα's block receptor-stimulated GTPase activity (9–11), and mastoparan, a positively charged peptide from wasp venom that is thought to activate G proteins by mimicking an intracellular loop of their receptors, can block the binding of $G\alpha_i$ C-terminal antibodies (11). A recent study using the *Drosophila* homolog of $G\alpha_S$ also suggests that residues very close to the C terminus are critical for coupling mammalian receptors to adenylate cyclase (12). These observations have been borne out in experiments with chimeric Gα's. Switching the C terminus of $G\alpha_S$ with that of $G\alpha_i$ results in the coupling of $G\alpha_i$ to stimulatory receptors (13). Similarly, inserting a fragment of $G\alpha_S$ into $G\alpha_i$ close to its C terminus results in $G\alpha_i$'s stimulating adenylate cyclase (14). Additional chimeric studies have pinpointed a region close to the N terminus of Gα's that might be involved in its interaction with β and/or γ subunits (14). The latter result is in agreement with earlier biochemical data (15). The α subunits of G_i and G_o are N-terminally myristoylated (16). This lipid modification is required for membrane association (17) and also for the efficient interaction of α subunits with the βγ dimer (18).

The G protein β and γ subunits are normally considered a single entity (the βγ dimer), as they require denaturing conditions for separation and coexpression for stability (19, 20). β subunits are 35–36 kDa and γ subunits are less than 10 kDa (see Ref. 2). Multiple forms of each subunit have been identified and there is indication that G protein–oligomer combinations differ between tissues (21). Having a variety of α, β, and γ combinations may increase the possible functional diversity of G proteins. The βγ dimer is essential for receptor–Gα interactions (22–24), but it is not yet clear whether this is due to a requirement for direct binding to the receptor. The βγ dimer appears hydrophobic in nature and can anchor Gα subunits to the plasma membrane (25). Neither the β nor the γ subunit has extensive hydrophobic sequence. However, the γ subunit is isoprenylated (for biochemical details see "C-Terminal Processing"), and this lipid attachment appears to be essential for βγ function (20). More active signaling roles for the βγ dimer have been postulated, particularly based on genetic analysis in yeast which suggests that the βγ dimer transduces the signal in response to mating pheromones (26). There is also evidence, albeit controversial, that the βγ dimer directly or indirectly regulates K^+ channels and phospholipase A_2 activity in mammalian cells (see Ref. 2).

GTP Cycle

G protein activity is regulated by cycling between GTP- and GDP-bound forms. G proteins are normally in the GDP-bound state under resting conditions; however, the activation of receptors by agonist binding results in stimulation of nucleotide exchange on Gα. This causes the activation of α subunits and, at least *in vitro*, the concomitant separation of Gα from the βγ dimer. Activated αGTP can then stimulate effector ion channels or enzymes until the intrinsic GTPase activity converts it back to the GDP-bound state. The αGDP then reassociates with the βγ dimer and is ready to undergo another cycle of receptor activation. G protein biochemistry and function have been described in more detail elsewhere (2, 5–7).

Neutrophil G Proteins

Pertussis Toxin-Sensitive G Proteins

There is considerable evidence to suggest that the effects of chemoattractant receptors are mediated through oligomeric G proteins (for reviews see Refs. 27 and 28). The majority of the biochemical responses elicited by chemoattractants (e.g., activation of phospholipases A_2, C, and D and mobilization of intracellular Ca^{2+}) are those normally associated with G protein activation (29). These effects are blocked by pretreatment of the cells with pertussis toxin, suggesting the involvement of G_i and/or G_o (30, 31). Further, the sensitivity of chemoattractant binding to its cognate receptor is modulated by guanine nucleotides (32, 33). The receptors for formylated peptides (34–36), C5a (37, 38), and platelet-activating factor (39) have recently been cloned and, as expected, have a predicted seven membrane-spanning domain structure, analogous to other G protein-coupled receptors (40). The kinetics of receptor–G protein coupling are described in Chapter 1 of this volume.

There are two $G\alpha$ proteins ADP-ribosylated by pertussis toxin in neutrophil membranes that are closely related to $G\alpha_i$ types 2 and 3, as determined by mapping of proteolytic digests, peptide sequencing, and immunoblotting (see Refs. 28 and 41). These data are supported by the identification of mRNAs for these two proteins in cDNA libraries made from differentiated HL-60 cells (42, 43). No $G\alpha_{i\text{-}1}$ or $G\alpha_o$ proteins or mRNAs have been detected in these cells. The major pertussis toxin substrate in neutrophils "$G\alpha_n$" is $G\alpha_{i\text{-}2}$. It is five to 10 times more abundant than $G\alpha_{i\text{-}3}$ and represents approximately 3% of membrane protein (44). Unlike $G\alpha_{i\text{-}3}$ and a 45-kDa form of $G\alpha_S$, the expression of $G\alpha_{i\text{-}2}$ is significantly increased upon myeloid differentiation of the HL-60 cells (41). G_i proteins have been found to copurify through several chromatographic steps with both formyl peptide (45) and C5a (46) receptors. Proteolytic digestion suggested that the major $G\alpha_i$ protein coupled to the formyl peptide receptor was $G\alpha_{i\text{-}2}$ (45). However, Gierschik *et al.* (47) have suggested that formyl peptide receptors are coupled to both forms of $G\alpha_i$. Cholera toxin is normally associated with the ADP ribosylation of $G\alpha_S$, not $G\alpha_i$, but in the presence of chemoattractant, it is possible to covalently modify receptor-coupled $G\alpha_i$ with cholera toxin. A likely explanation for this phenomenon is that the target arginine residue in the nucleotide binding pocket of $G\alpha_i$ is exposed to cholera toxin only during nucleotide exchange (when no nucleotide is bound). Treatment of neutrophil membranes with cholera toxin plus f–Met–Leu–Phe in the absence of guanine nucleotides resulted in the ADP ribosylation of two proteins that comigrate with HL-60 cell pertussis toxin substrates $G\alpha_{i\text{-}2}$ and $G\alpha_{i\text{-}3}$ (47, 48). Katada and colleagues (49) have also suggested that the formyl peptide receptor couples to functionally distinct forms of $G\alpha_{i\text{-}2}$.

The ability of chemoattractant receptors to interact with G proteins has recently been directly demonstrated for both C5a and formyl peptide receptors. Rollins *et al.* (50) isolated the C5a receptor using an affinity matrix and observed that three major proteins were specifically and stoichiometrically eluted. One of these proteins was the C5a receptor, as determined by photoaffinity labeling, whereas the other two, 40- and 36-kDa, proteins were shown to be G protein α and β subunits, respectively, by pertussis toxin labeling and reaction with α- and β-specific antisera. Jesaitis *et al.* (51) had previously shown that [^{125}I]f–Met–Leu–Phe–Leu–SASD [sulfosuccinimidyl 2-(*p*-azidosalicylamido) ethyl-1,3′-dithiopropionate]-labeled formyl peptide receptor could be extracted from neutrophil membranes in a form with a sedimentation coefficient of 7 S.

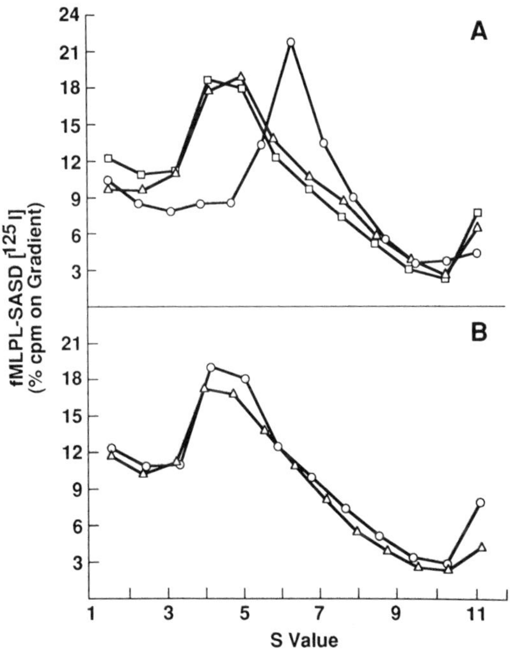

FIGURE 1

Physical association of the formyl peptide receptor with G_i. The[^{125}I]fMLPL–SASD-labeled formyl peptide receptor forms a 7 S complex with pure G_i protein. (A) The "basal" receptor (Δ) migrates as a 4 S form, but when constituted with brain G_i, it shifts to a 7 S form (○). Addition of 10 μ*M* GTPγS uncouples receptor from the G protein, yielding the 4 S form (□). (B) The G_i protein stoichiometrically ADP-ribosylated by pertussis toxin can no longer form a 7 S complex with receptor (○). Δ Basal receptor. Analysis is described in Ref. 52.

The receptor could be converted to a 4 S form by treatment with guanine nucleotides, suggesting that the 7 S form represented a complex of receptor and G protein. In collaboration with Jesaitis and associates (52), we have subsequently shown that the 4 S form of the receptor can be directly converted to sediment at 7 S by reconstitution with purified neutrophil or brain G_i (Fig. 1). This shift to the 7 S form is prevented by pertussis toxin-catalyzed ADP ribosylation of G_i and is sensitive to guanine nucleotides. The assignment of the endogenous 7 S species as a complex between the receptor and the G protein is thus confirmed.

Activation of phospholipase C and, more recently, phospholipase D in neutrophils has been shown to be sensitive to guanine nucleotides, suggesting G protein regulation (53, 54). It was recently reported that formyl peptide-stimulated diacylglycerol and phosphatidate generation shows differential sensitivity to inhibition by pertussis toxin treatment of cells (55). Thus, it is possible that $G\alpha_{i\text{-}2}$ and $G\alpha_{i\text{-}3}$ couple formyl peptide receptors to different phospholipases. Phospholipase activation is the topic of Chapter 3 in this volume.

Pertussis Toxin-Insensitive G Proteins

While, in general, the responses of neutrophils to chemoattractants are sensitive to the pertussis toxin treatment of cells, several non-pertussis toxin-sensitive events have been observed, including purinergic stimulation of phospholipase C (56) and elevation of intracellular free calcium by platelet-activating factor (27). These data suggest that G proteins other than $G\alpha_i$ may exist in phagocytic cells. Recently, new classes of $G\alpha$ protein have been identified by the polymerase chain reaction (PCR) and subsequent cloning (57, 58). These proteins, as well as $G\alpha_Z$ (59), lack the cysteine residue that is ADP-ribosylated in $G\alpha_i$ and have several other key features that warrant their being categorized as a family separate from $G\alpha_i$. Most notably, the GAGES (single-letter amino acid code) sequence in the nucleotide binding region closest to the N terminus of the PCR-derived clones (see Fig. 2) is converted to GTGES (57). One of these α subunits, G_q, appears to be the pertussis toxin-insensitive G protein that couples receptors to phospholipase C in cells of (mostly) nonhematopoietic origin (60) and, along with $G\alpha_{11}$, is ubiquitously expressed (58). Two other $G\alpha$s ($G\alpha$-types 15 and 16) are expressed preferentially in leukocytes (61) and may be responsible for pertussis toxin-insensitive signaling. The ability of chemoattractant receptors to interact with such G proteins has not yet been demonstrated.

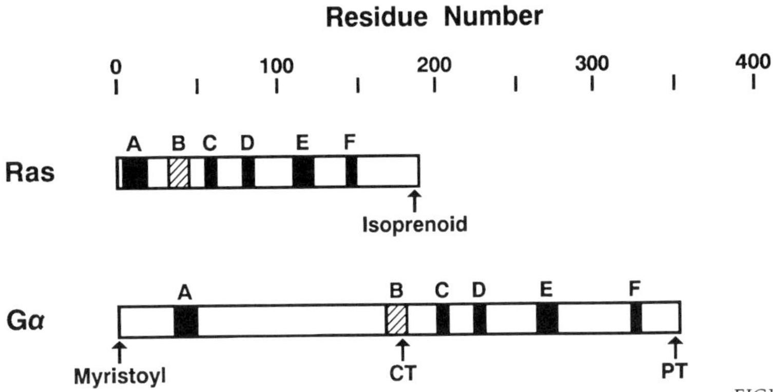

FIGURE 2

Nucleotide binding regions and sites of posttranslational modification of Ras and G*α*. Regions of Ras that are involved in the binding and/or hydrolysis of GTP (A–F) are shown, along with homologous regions in the $G\alpha_i$ sequence. The hatched region shows the putative effector binding domain of Ras and the equivalent region in G*α*. CT and PT, Arg-179 and Cys-351 that are ADP-ribosylated by cholera and pertussis toxins, respectively; myristoyl, site of myristoylation of $G\alpha_i$; isoprenoid, site of farnesylation or geranylgeranylation of LMWGs.

Low-Molecular-Weight G Proteins

LMWG Subfamilies

In addition to the oligomeric G proteins, there is a rapidly growing superfamily of LMWGs being identified by protein purification, immunological, and recombinant technologies (3, 4, 62, 63). This superfamily currently consists of approximately 40 monomeric proteins in the range of 18–28 kDa. Based on primary sequence, they have been subdivided into three major families.

The *ras* oncogene products were the original LMWGs to be discovered and are the most extensively studied. The 21-kDa Ha-, Ki-, and N-Ras are believed to be involved in growth factor-mediated signal transduction, either by modulating known second messenger systems or by acting through a novel pathway(s) (64–70). The Ras family of LMWGs consists of an additional seven proteins that have approximately 50% homology with

Ras. These include R-Ras (71), Ral A and B (72), and the Rap subfamily (73–75). The functions of the former are unknown, while the Rap proteins are discussed with respect to antagonism of Ras action and phagocytic function(s) in "Regulation of GTP Hydrolysis" and "G Protein Regulation of Oxidant Production in Neutrophils." There are four Raps: 1A and 1B, which are 95% homologous, and 2 and 2B, which are also very similar to each other (90% homology) and 70% homologous with Rap1A. Rap1A was independently cloned by several groups (73, 76, 77) and is also known as Krev-1 (78) and smg p21 (79).

The second group of LMWGs is the Rho family, which currently consists of seven mammalian members: RhoA–C (80), Rac1 and 2 (81), and G25K 1 and 2 (82, 83). These proteins have approximately 30% homology with Ha-Ras, mostly confined to regions involved in the binding of guanine nucleotides. The Rho, and possibly also the Rac, proteins are characterized by their ability to be ADP-ribosylated by *Clostridium botulinum* exoenzyme C_3 (81, 84, 85). The site of ADP ribosylation (Asp-41) is in an equivalent position in Rho as the Arg-201 of $G\alpha_S$ that is ADP-ribosylated by cholera toxin (85). However, although cholera toxin activates $G\alpha_S$ by inhibiting its GTPase activity, ADP ribosylation of Rho does not have such an effect (84). Microinjection of cells with *C. botulinum* exoenzyme C_3 or with a mutant Rho protein affected their morphology and induced the dissolution of actin filaments (86, 87). This suggests that Rho proteins play some role in cytoskeletal organization. Interestingly, expression of the Rac2 protein is restricted to cells of hematopoietic origin (81, 88).

The third group of LMWGs includes the Rab proteins. These proteins share homology with Ypt1, a yeast protein that has been implicated in vesicular trafficking (89). Recent studies in mammalian cells suggest that the Rabs play similar roles in both endocytic and exocytic pathways (reviewed in Ref. 90). Twelve Rab clones have been reported so far (91); however, at least as many additional sequences have been identified, suggesting that the roles of these proteins may be more diverse. The key structural features of the Rab proteins are the absence of a glycine residue at the equivalent of position 12 in Ras and the possession of a Cys–Cys or Cys–X–Cys C-terminal sequence.

The ARF (ADP ribosylation factor) and related GTP binding proteins may be considered as a fourth family in the LMWG grouping. These proteins differ somewhat from the Ras, Rho, and Rab proteins in terms of their overall sequence homology, their lack of a C-terminal cysteine (and thus isoprenylation), and their myristoylation at a glycine residue at position 2. The ARF proteins have been shown to be necessary components of the Golgi apparatus intracellular protein transport pathway (180).

LMWG Structure–Function Relationship

Guanine Nucleotide Binding Site

Four principal domains of homology exist between all G proteins that are colinear within each primary sequence (regions A, C, D, and E in Fig. 2). Indeed, based on the X-ray crystallographic data available for Ras and EF-Tu and the predicted tertiary structures of Gα's, it is likely that all G proteins are folded in a similar fashion (92, 93). The generation of structural mutants of Ras suggested that these regions are important for the binding and hydrolysis of GTP. Now that the three-dimensional structure of Ras has been determined, it has been confirmed that the NKXD (corresponding to residues 116–119 of Ras) and SAK (146–148) sequences are involved in binding the guanine ring and that GXGXXGKS (10–17) and DTAGQE (59–61) are involved in binding and hydrolyzing, respectively, the γ-phosphate of GTP (92, 94) (see Fig. 2). X-Ray crystallographic data show that the highly conserved residue Thr-35 also interacts with the guanine nucleotide (94). Three-dimensional studies have revealed two key areas of Ras that occupy different conformations in the GTP- and GDP-bound states. These are located between residues 30–38 and 60–76 (92, 95) and are discussed in relation to interaction with regulatory and effector molecules in the following sections.

Regulation of GTP Hydrolysis

The intrinsic GTPase activity of the LMWGs (~0.01 min^{-1} is generally much slower than that of oligomeric G proteins. However, in 1987 a GTPase-activating protein (GAP) was identified that stimulates the GTPase activity of Ras some 200-fold (96). GAPs have since been identified for the Rho (97) and Rap1 families (98, 99) and Rab3A (smg p25A) (100). The NF-1 gene product, responsible for the genetic disorder neurofibromatosis, has also been identified as a Ras GAP (101).

Point mutations between residues 32 and 40 of Ras were found to block the ability of GAP to stimulate and, in some cases, even interact with Ras (102–104). These same mutants had previously been shown to block the transforming activity of Ras, leading to speculation that the 32–40 region is the site of interaction of Ras with an effector molecule (105, 106). This implies that GAP functions as a mediator of Ras action and as its terminator. In support of the role of GAP as a negative regulator/off switch for Ras, overexpression of GAP in fibroblasts has been shown to attenuate Ras-induced transformation (107). Further, inhibition of GAP activity through a protein kinase C-mediated pathway apparently results in Ras activation in T lymphocytes (108). The likelihood that GAP is also the effector of Ras action is nonetheless supported by several pieces of evidence: (1) Oncogenic forms of Ras, whose GTPase activity is not stimulated by GAP, still bind tightly to it (103). (2) Microinjection of a mutant yeast Ras, which has high affinity for GAP but cannot localize to the plasma membrane, into frog oocytes prevented *ras*-induced germinal vesicle breakdown. This effect could be overcome by addition of exogenous GAP (109). (3) Recombinant GAP blocks the carbachol-stimulated opening of K^+ channels on patch-clamped atrial cell membranes (69). This effect of GAP only occurred in the presence of RasGTP, suggesting that a RasGTP–GAP complex sends a transient signal prior to self-termination. Interestingly, a region of $G\alpha_S$ showing sequence homology with the effector domain of Ras is closely followed by sequence similar to part of the catalytic domain of GAP (110). Thus, the higher intrinsic GTPase activity of oligomeric versus LMWG proteins may be due to the built-up GAP region of the former proteins.

The site(s) of interaction of GAPs with other LMWGs has yet to be determined. However, Rap1A, which has sequence identity with Ras between residues 32 and 44, interacts with *ras*GAP. RapGTP has a considerably higher affinity for *ras*GAP than Ras (111, 112), although the GTPase activity of wild-type Rap is not stimulated by *ras*GAP (76, 112). Regions flanking the effector sequence have been reported to dictate the GAP specificity of these two LMWGs (113); however, a Thr-61–Gln Rap1 mutant is partially responsive to *ras*GAP (unpublished observations; 112, 114), suggesting that the Thr-61 residue of Rap1 is also critical in dictating GAP specificity. Rap1A has been shown to reverse the phenotype characteristic of Ras-transformed murine fibroblasts (78). Also, Rap1B was recently shown to block Ras-induced germinal vesicle breakdown of frog oocytes (115). The basis for this function is anticipated to be the antagonism of Ras action by interaction with *ras*GAP. In support of this notion, we have recently demonstrated that Rap1A–GTPγS, but not a Thr-35–A1a Rap1A mutant, will prevent *ras*GAP from blocking atrial K^+ channel opening. This effect of Rap1A can be overcome by adding more Ras or *ras*GAP to the system (116). A recent report suggests that the yeast YptGAP is also an intracellular target of the Rab-related Ypt1 protein and that it interacts with a region equivalent to the Ras effector domain (117). This is consistent with data showing that peptides representing the effector domain of Rab block its ability to transport proteins from the endoplasmic reticulum to the Golgi apparatus (118).

Regulation of Nucleotide Exchange

The Ras-neutralizing monoclonal antibody Y13-259 has been shown to bind to a region of Ras between residues 63 and 73 (105, 119). While

Y13-259 does not prevent binding of nucleotide, it inhibits the exchange between bound nucleotide and that in solution (120, 121). This finding, along with the significant change in conformation of this region between the GTP- and GDP-bound forms of the protein (92), has led to speculation that this is the site of regulation by a guanine nucleotide exchange factor. This region of Ras is dispensable for transformation (122), consistent with its playing a role in signal input, rather than effector function. Exchange factors [or, perhaps more correctly, guanine nucleotide dissociation stimulators (GDSs) that promote the release of GDP so that the more abundant cytosolic GTP can bind] have been partially purified for Ras (123–125). Activation of Ras in T cells has been reported to occur through inhibition of GAP activity, the GDSs apparently being constitutively active (108). Thus, caution should be taken in drawing analogy between the roles of LMWG GDSs and G protein-coupled receptors in the activation of LMWGs. However, the *Saccharomyces cerevisiae* Ras GDS [the CDC25 gene product (126)] is under regulation and the C-terminal (catalytic) domain of the related SDC25 stimulates the formation of RasGTP when introduced into mammalian cells (127). This supports the notion that a GDS can activate Ras and that at least the yeast GDS homologs are not constitutively active, but rather have regulatory domains. A cytosolic GDS has also been identified for Rap1 (128) as well as GDIs (nucleotide dissociation inhibitors) for Rho (129) and Rab3A [smg p25a (130)]. The Rho and Rab GDIs have been cloned (131, 132) and bear weak homology with CDC25.

The amount of mammalian GDS or GDI required to modulate nucleotide exchange *in vitro* is very high compared to the catalytic amount of GAP needed to stimulate GTP hydrolysis (128, 130). This may be due to the loss of a regulatory element upon purification. Several recent reports by Takai and colleagues have demonstrated that both GDIs and GDSs promote the translocation of LMWGs from the membrane (133–135) and, at least in the case of Rap1, stoichiometric amounts of GDS are required (133). The requirement for stoichiometric amounts of Rab proteins and nucleotide dissociation regulators to promote membrane translocation and/or nucleotide exchange would be compatible with the apparent role of Rabs in directing vesicular traffic (90, 136). Being converted to the GTP-bound form when leaving, for example, an acceptor vesicle membrane or being maintained in a GDP-bound state by interaction with a GDI until back on a donor membrane might drive the system unidirectionally. The integrity of the LMWG C terminus is essential for the action of nucleotide dissociation regulators (135, 137), suggesting that this region might be a point of interaction between the two molecules. Since the C terminus is involved in the membrane localization of LMWGs (see the following section), this observation might explain how GDSs and GDIs promote translocation from the plasma membrane.

Posttranslational Modification

C-Terminal Processing. A feature common to Ras, Rho, and some Rab family members, in addition to several other mammalian proteins, including the nuclear lamins and G proteins γ subunits, is the C-terminal sequence CAAX (where C is cysteine, A is aliphatic, and X represents almost any amino acid) (138). Mutation of this region, for example, by introducing a Cys→Ser mutation in the Ras or Rap1A –CAAX, prevents a series of posttranslational modifications and, subsequently, the membrane localization and biology of the molecules (139, 140). The cysteine residue is the site of prenylation by a 15-carbon farnesyl group from farnesyl pyrophosphate in the case of Ras (141–143) (see Fig. 3), or the 20-carbon geranylgeranyl for Rap1A (140) (Figs. 3 and 4) and most other LMWGs, including Rap1B (144), Racs (145), G25K (146), and Rho (147).

Prenylation is a signal for the proteolytic removal of the AAX residues, exposing the free COOH group of the prenylated cysteine to a methyltransferase (148, 149; for reviews see Refs. 138 and 150). The γ subunit of retinal transducin is processed by farnesyl and methyl groups similarly to Ras (151), whereas the other Gγ''s are geranylgeranylated (152). The choice of lipid is dictated by the individual AAX sequence (150, 153); however, the physiological implication of a C15 versus C20 modification is currently unclear. The C terminus of Rap1A is able to support transformation by H-ras in a Ras–Rap chimera (140). Thus, at least some geranylgeranylated Ras must still find its way to the correct subcellular location (i.e., the plasma membrane). It is now clear that separate enzymes are involved in transferring C15 and C20 isoprene groups to LMWGs (147, 153, 154). Further, a novel C20 prenyltransferase(s) is responsible for modifying the C terminus of the Rab proteins that have Cys–Cys or Cys–X–Cys sequences (154).

Addition of a farnesyl group to the C terminus of Ras increases its hydrophobicity such that it partitions into the detergent phase at a Triton X-114/water interface (141). However, without subsequent truncation and methylation of the protein, it will not bind efficiently to membranes (149). Truncation presumably enables the prenyl group to more effectively integrate into the membrane, assisted by the reduction of charge by methylation. Although each of these processing events is essential, it is not sufficient to promote the membrane localization of LMWGs. Ha-, Ki-Ras4A-, and N-Ras (141) and, presumably, Rap2 (155) rely on the additional palmitoylation of upstream cysteine residues [182 and 184 in the

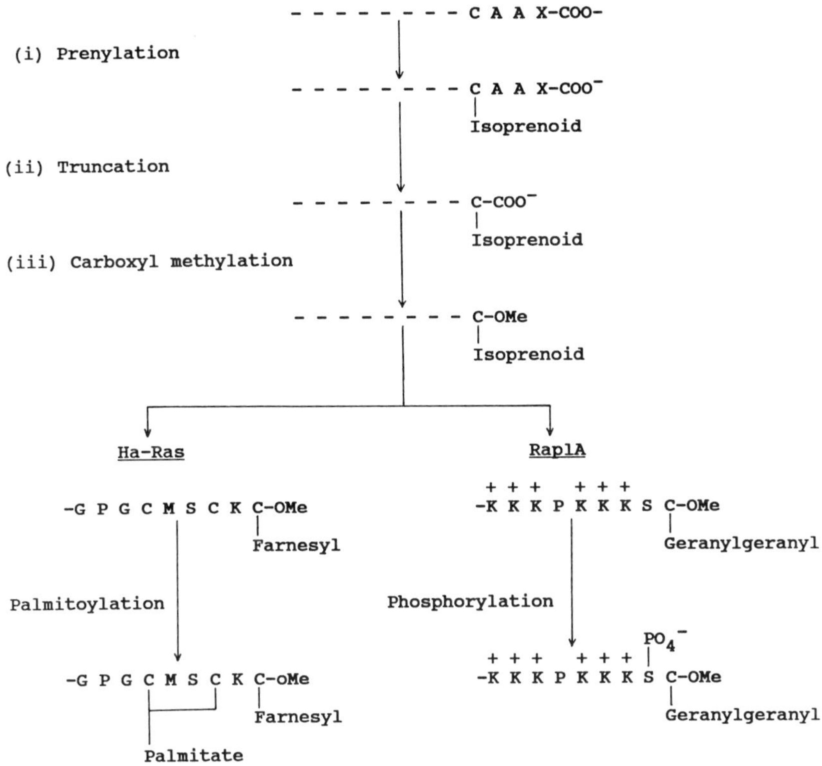

FIGURE 3

C-Terminal processing pathways for Ha-Ras and Rap1A. The first step in the processing of CAAX-containing peptides is the addition of farnesol in the case of Ras or geranylgeranyl for Rap1A and other LMWGs. Addition of this lipid moiety signals proteolytic cleavage of the –AAX residues (step ii) and methylation of the now C-terminal cysteine (step iii). These processing events allow the subsequent palmitoylation of Ha-Ras on upstream cysteine residue(s). Other LMWGs have positively charged C-terminal sequences that assist in membrane association (see text). Rap1A is phosphorylated by cAMP-dependent protein kinase (PK-A) on a serine residue adjacent to the processed cysteine. Although a peptide representing the unprocessed Rap1A C terminus is a substrate for PK-A (169), we found that unprocessed Rap1A is not as readily phosphorylated as the 22-kDa isoprenylated protein (unpublished observations).

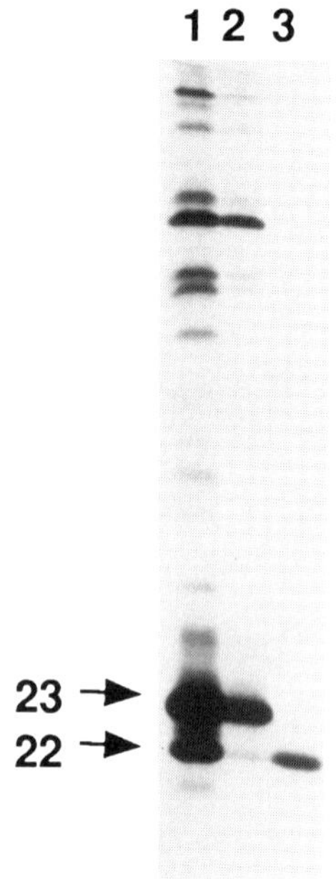

FIGURE 4

Isoprenylation and processing of Rap1A. Sf9 cells infected with *rap*1A-containing baculovirus were labeled with the isoprenoid precursor mevalonic acid or with [^{35}S]methionine for 24 hr. Lanes 1 and 2 show the incorporation of [^{35}S]methionine into Sf9 cell proteins in the absence (lane 1) or presence (lane 2) of compactin, an inhibitor of endogenous mevalonate (and consequently) isoprenoid biosynthesis. Both 23-kDa precursor and 22-kDa mature protein are present in lane 1, but, in the presence of compactin, the 23-kDa precursor form predominates. Lane 3 shows the incorporation of [^{3}H]mevalonic acid into only the 22-kDa processed form of Rap1A. Following immunoprecipitation of Rap1A and extraction of the lipid, it was found to represent a 20-carbon isoprenoid (see Ref. 140 for details).

case of Ha-Ras (141)]. Other proteins, including K-Ras4B and Rap1A, have a high density of basic, mostly lysine, residues close to their C termini (see Fig. 3). These apparently promote membrane localization in place of palmitate, through ionic interaction with negatively charged phospholipids (143, 156).

The Gγ subunits do not have upstream cysteine or polylysine regions (Gγ C termini have a net charge of +2 compared with +6 for Ki-Ras4B and Rap1A). Therefore, it is not clear how the βγ dimer associates with the plasma membrane. Since the yeast α mating factor, processed similarly to Ras, has a cell surface receptor [homologous with G protein-coupled receptors (157)], there is speculation that a similar entity might exist for Ras on the inner surface of the plasma membrane. The requirement for hydrophobic palmitate or the highly charged polylysine, which could bind negatively charged phospholipids (e.g., polyphosphoinositides), for membrane binding suggests that receptors may not be necessary. However, the demonstration of receptors for the myristoylated protein $p60^{src}$ (158) and the effect of the Ki-Ras4B C terminus on the activity of several key membrane-bound enzymes (159) suggest that this possibility should not be ruled out.

Carboxyl methylation of unidentified LMWGs in macrophage membranes has been reported to be sensitive to guanine nucleotides (160). This phenomenon has been shown for both Rap1A (unpublished observations) and 1B (161). Since methylation is necessary for efficient membrane localization of Ras, the nucleotide-bound state of Rap1 might affect its subcellular localization.

Phosphorylation. Several of the LMWGs have been reported to serve as substrates for protein kinases, both *in vitro* and *in vivo*. Rap1A and 1B are stoichiometrically phosphorylated by cAMP-dependent protein kinase (162–164), and increased phosphorylation of Rap1B has been demonstrated in platelets upon elevation of cAMP (162, 164). We have similarly shown that Rap1A can be phosphorylated in permeabilized neutrophils by addition of cAMP (165), and recombinant Rap1A is phosphorylated in response to forskolin when expressed in murine fibroblasts (unpublished observations). A protein recognized by Rap1-specific antisera (thought to be Rap1A) is phosphorylated in response to the treatment of HL-60 cells with isoproterenol or prostaglandin E_1 (165). Phosphorylation of Rap1B has been reported to induce its translocation from the plasma membrane to the cytosol (164). In contrast, Rap1B moves to the platelet cytoskeleton in response to treatment with thrombin or the calcium ionophore, A23187 (166). Rap1B is also phosphorylated *in vitro* by the neuronal Ca^{2+}/calmodulin-dependent protein kinase (167). Phosphorylation of Rap1B has been reported to increase its sensitivity to GDS activity (168). However, the physiological significance of these events is as yet unclear.

We have determined the site of phosphorylation of Rap1A to be Ser-180 (165). This residue is adjacent to the geranylgeranylated Cys-181 (see Fig. 3). The negative phosphate might prevent efficient intercalation of the isoprenoid group into the membrane (similarly to an unmethylated COO^- terminus) or disrupt the ionic interaction between polylysines and phospholipids/receptor protein. A serine two residues upstream of Cys-

181 is also the site of phosphorylation of Rap1B (168, 169). The Rab2 and 4 proteins were recently reported to serve as substrates for the cell cycle kinase, $p34^{cdc2}$ (170). The consensus sequence for this kinase is also close to the C terminus. Although Ki-Ras4B was phosphorylated with low stoichiometry *in vitro* (171), it was reported to be a substrate for protein kinase C *in vivo* (172). Since this effect was not seen with the alternately spliced Ki-Ras4A, Ser-181 and -171, four and 15 residues upstream of the CAAX, are the likely sites of phosphorylation. Other LMWGs including RhoA, Ral, and Rab8 are potential substrates for kinases due to having phosphorylation consensus sequences in their basic C termini. Also, G25K has been shown to be phosphorylated on a tyrosine residue(s) by the epidermal growth factor receptor (173).

Whether the role of phosphorylation is to modulate processing, neutralize the basic domain required for membrane binding, or regulate interaction with GDSs, GDIs, or other molecules remains to be determined.

LMWGs in Neutrophils

Considering the proposed roles of LMWGs in cellular signaling, vesicular transport, and cytoskeletal organization, one might expect these proteins to be abundant in phagocytic cells. We have purified several LMWGs from human neutrophil membranes, including Rap1A and two unidentified proteins termed G24K and G26K (163, 174, 175). An additional membrane-bound LMWG that comigrates with Rap1A on polyacrylamide gels and is ADP-ribosylated by *C. botulinum* exoenzyme C_3 has been partially purified and is possibly a form of Rac or Rho (81, 85, 175). Another C_3 substrate has also been isolated from neutrophil cytosol that contains a sequence identical to RhoA (unpublished observations). A role for a G protein in the assembly of actin microfilaments in neutrophils has been suggested by work from several laboratories (176–179). These studies demonstrated that GTP and nonhydrolyzable GTP analogs could induce actin polymerization in permeabilized cells. This effect was blocked by GDPβS and was insensitive to pertussis and cholera toxins. Further, stimulation of actin assembly was not dependent on phospholipase C activation. Sarndahl *et al.* (176) have also provided evidence that the association of *N*-formyl peptide–chemoattractant receptor complexes with the Triton X-100-insoluble cytoskeleton might be regulated by a pertussis toxin-insensitive G protein. While it has not been shown that the GTP-binding component in these phenomena is an LMWG, the recently demonstrated effects of Rho activation and *C. botulinum* exoenzyme C_3 on actin assembly (86, 87) and the association of Rap1B with the cytoskeleton in platelets upon stimulation by thrombin (166) are suggestive in this regard.

Several other LMWGs have been demonstrated in neutrophils by [^{32}P]GTP-blotting and immunoblotting, purification, and cloning. For example, we have identified ADP ribosylation factor (ARF), a GTP-binding protein required for cholera toxin-catalyzed ADP ribosylation of G_S and recently associated with the Golgi apparatus (180), by blotting neutrophil fractions with ARF antisera (unpublished observations). A *ral* clone was isolated from a cDNA library from differentiated HL-60 cells (181) and might represent G26K. Using specific antisera, the abundance of Rabs 1, 2, 4, and 6 has been shown to increase upon differentiation of U937 and HL-60 cells along the myeloid pathway (182). These proteins were located mostly in membrane fractions, partially in the cytosol, but not, as might have been expected, in the phagocytic (azurophil or specific) granules. Approximately 15 neutrophil LMWGs were indicated in a recent study by Phillips *et al.* (183). Although few were identified, subcellular fractionation demonstrated several potentially novel LMWGs in phagocytic granules. However, some caution must be taken when considering the subcellular distribution of LMWGs. For example, different patterns of *C. botulinum* exoenzyme C_3 substrates have been found by us and by Phillips *et al.* (183). These differences may be attributable to the method of cell lysis or the degree of priming of the neutrophils upon isolation.

An as yet unidentified G protein, G_e has been described by Gomperts, Cockcroft, and colleagues (184–186) in neutrophils and other cells. Their data clearly indicate that a GTP-dependent process, separate from that required for signal transduction, is involved in mediating stimulated secretion. GTP and its analogs stimulate secretion in permeabilized cells without elevation of the intracellular Ca^{2+} concentration and can enhance the responses to various secretagogues at low Ca^{2+} levels (186, 187). Oncogenic forms of Ras cause membrane ruffling and pinocytosis shortly after microinjection into fibroblasts and, when injected into mast cells, promote exocytic degranulation (188). These observations support the notion that Ras-related LMWGs are involved in exocytosis. This would be consistent with the apparently extensive role of Rab proteins in vesicular trafficking (90).

The HL-60 premyeloid leukemia cell line has been shown to have an activated *ras* gene; however, the level of Ras expression in HL-60 cells and human neutrophils is considerably lower than that of the other LMWGs that we have identified. This raises the question as to the role of Rap1A in these cells. If its role is to counteract or regulate Ras action, why is it expressed in such high abundance [0.2% of membrane protein (163, 165)] in a terminally differentiated cell containing little Ras? The abundance of the closely related Rap1B in platelets suggests that these proteins have specific functions in cells of hematopoietic origin. A possible role for Rap1A in neutrophils is discussed in the following sections.

G Protein Regulation of Oxidant Production in Neutrophils

Evidence for the Involvement of G Proteins in Oxidant Production

The activation of neutrophil oxidant formation via chemoattractant receptor-mediated mechanisms appears to involve G proteins at two levels. It is clear that chemoattractant receptor signaling involves a pertussis toxin-sensitive G protein which couples to the receptor and mediates activation of phospholipase C and, potentially, other phospholipases (see Refs. 28 and 31). The formation of intracellular mediators via these effector enzymes results in activation of the NADPH oxidase system by still undefined mechanisms. The stimulation of superoxide formation via chemoattractant receptors can thus be inhibited at the level of the receptor-generated signal by pertussis toxin-catalyzed ADP ribosylation of G_n.

It has become increasingly evident, however, that a G protein may be involved in regulating the NADPH oxidase at a level downstream of the receptor-initiated pathway. Using cell-free systems in which oxidase activity is stimulated by nonphysiological perturbants such as sodium dodecyl sulfate or high concentrations of arachidonic acid, numerous investigators have described the ability of nonhydrolyzable guanine nucleotides to enhance the activity of the NADPH oxidase (189–191). Complementing the observed stimulatory effects of guanine nucleotide triphosphate analogs, guanine nucleotide diphosphates (GDP and GDPβS) were found to inhibit oxidase activation in the cell-free system. The stimulatory effects of guanine nucleotides on NADPH oxidase activation have been reported in various permeabilized neutrophil preparations as well (192).

While these studies have implicated a guanine nucleotide-binding protein in the modulation of superoxide formation, they do not indicate a critical role for such a protein in this process. Since all of the cell-free systems utilized in the aforementioned studies require the addition of cytosol in order for activity to be observed, it seems obvious (at least in retrospect) that endogenous GTP would already be present in the assay system. In the one study in which pains were taken to remove cytosolic

GTP prior to testing (193), it was shown that there is actually an absolute requirement for GTP in order for activation of the NADPH oxidase to occur. These data strongly indicate that a GTP-binding component is an integral part of the NADPH oxidase system, and must be present in an activated (i.e., GTP-bound) form in order for superoxide formation to occur.

Studies with cell-free oxidase systems have demonstrated the requirement for both cytosolic and membrane-associated factors (194). Where is the subcellular location at which GTP acts? Several studies have suggested that this component might be membrane associated. Ligeti *et al.* (195) observed enhanced oxidase activation upon preincubation of membrane with GTPγS versus preincubation of cytosol with GTPγS. Similarly, Bolscher *et al.* (196) observed GTPγS effects predominantly at the membrane level, albeit in the presence of a cytosolic protein factor. However, these studies are also consistent with the functional effect of the relevant G protein being *mediated* at the level of the membrane. The majority of the studies which have attempted to localize the site of the GTPγS-binding component by GTPγS pretreatment of the relevant fractions have indicated that it resides in the cytosol. Indeed, several cytosolic factors have been implicated as the potential GTP-binding candidate, including the Soc I, NCF-3, and σ1 factors (196, 197). A definitive answer to this question will require purification and characterization of a G protein(s) which can be shown to be a required component in the oxidase system.

Gabig *et al.* (189) initially suggested that the action of GTPγS to stimulate the NADPH oxidase system was mediated via a pertussis toxin-insensitive G protein. As we have pointed out previously (28), such data are not particularly convincing, since GTPγS-mediated G protein activation is largely unaffected by pertussis toxin-catalyzed ADP ribosylation. Additionally, we have demonstrated the existence of cytosolic $G\alpha_n$ subunits which are not associated with βγ subunits, rendering them insensitive to the action of pertussis toxin, which acts on the heteromeric (αβγ) complex (44). The demonstrated existence in myeloid cells of (heterotrimeric) G protein α subunits which lack pertussis toxin ADP ribosylation sites (61) also complicates the situation.

Are there any data at this point which indicate that the relevant oxidase-associated G protein is an LMWG, rather than a heteromeric G protein? One indication that this is the case comes from work by Gabig *et al.* (198). In this study they showed that preincubation of a cytosolic fraction with GTPγS under conditions of low Mg^{2+} concentration allowed effective activation of the putative oxidase-associated G protein to occur. Such an effect would be consistent with the properties of the Ras-like LMWGs which readily exchange guanine nucleotides at low Mg^{2+} concentrations (163). A second indication that an LMWG might be involved comes from recent data obtained in our laboratory which show that it is possible to block activation of the NADPH oxidase by treating HL-60 cells with compactin (215). Compactin blocks the posttranslational prenylation of LMWGs by inhibiting the enzyme HMG-CoA reductase, thereby blocking mevalonate and subsequent isoprenoid syntheses. We find that treating HL-60 cells differentiated with dimethyl sulfoxide with concentrations of compactin (0.4–10 μM) that can be shown to inhibit the prenylation of endogenous Rap1 protein totally blocks the ability of the cells to generate superoxide anion in response to either f–Met–Leu–Phe or phorbol myristate acetate. The cells are still viable and differentiate "normally" in terms of their ability to express the N-formyl peptide receptor. These data are supportive of a role of LMWGs in the process of NADPH oxidase activation.

Rap1A binds to the Cytochrome b_{558} Component of the NADPH Oxidase System

Currently, the Rap1A protein of human neutrophils is a candidate for being an LMWG which might regulate the NADPH oxidase system. The initial indication for this came when Quinn *et al.* (77) observed the coisolation during conventional purification of the cytochrome *b* of a 22-kDa protein (distinct from the cytochrome *b* α subunit) which had an amino-terminal amino acid sequence identical to that of Rap1. Evidence that this was not merely a coincident purification (since separation did occur at the final sucrose gradient step) was provided by their observation that a similar 22-kDa protein present in partially purified cytochrome *b* preparations would bind to anticytochrome 91-kDa or 22-kDa subunit–antibody beads. These data suggested that a Rap1-like protein could interact with the cytochrome. However, since other proteins can be shown to be present in these partially purified cytochrome *b* preparations (199), a direct interaction with the cytochrome *b* itself could not be concluded.

Our laboratory, in conjunction with M. T. Quinn and A. J. Jesaitis, has recently investigated the ability of highly purified preparations of Rap1A and cytochrome b_{558} to form complexes *in vitro* (200). As shown in Fig. 5, we are able to observe the formation of a complex between GTPγS-bound Rap1A and cytochrome *b*, as assessed by a shift in the apparent size of the [^{35}S]GTPγS-labeled Rap1A upon gel filtration analysis (Fig. 5). Several controls indicate that this is a Rap-specific interaction, including the inability of GTPγS-bound H-Ras to form such a complex and the requirement for active (nondenatured) Rap1A for complexation to occur. Additionally, GTPγS-bound Rap1A does not form a complex with G protein $\beta\gamma$ subunits under similar conditions. The latter data indicate that this interaction is not

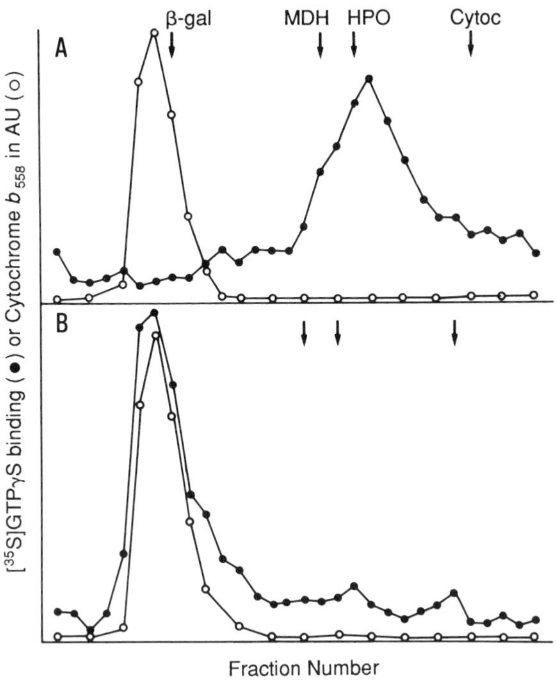

FIGURE 5

Physical association between Rap1A and cytochrome b_{558}. The ability of Rap1A protein to form an *in vitro* complex with cytochrome *b* was analyzed by gel filtration. (A) Cytochrome *b* (○) and [^{35}S]GTPγS-bound Rap1A (●) migrate as distinct molecular species when chromatographed separately. After preincubation together, the Rap1A [^{35}S]GTPγS associates with and coelutes with cytochrome *b*. Arrows indicate the positions at which the markers β-galactosidase (β-gal), malate dehydrogenase (MDH), horseradish peroxidase (HPO), and cytochrome C (Cyto) elute. AU, arbitrary units. Further details can be obtained in Ref. 200.

a nonspecific association of Rap1A with hydrophobic membrane-associated proteins.

Is Rap1A the "Oxidase Regulatory Protein" Involved in the Stimulatory Effects of Guanine Nucleotide?

While it seems clear that Rap1A can interact with the cytochrome *b*, the significance of this interaction is not yet clear is in terms of NADPH oxidase activation. We have as yet observed no ability of Rap1A protein to modulate the activity of the cell-free NADPH oxidase system (unpublished observations). We also find Rap1A to be totally absent (at our levels of detectability) from neutrophil cytosol, using a variety of Rap1-specific antisera generated in our laboratory (165). This absence from cytosol would seem to preclude Rap1A from being the protein responsible for GTPγS effects on the oxidase, which appear to be resident in the cytosol, as discussed earlier.

On the other hand, a role for Rap1A in regulating the oxidase is attractive because of the ability of Rap1A to serve as a substrate for cAMP-dependent protein kinase (163, 165). Agents that elevate neutrophil cAMP have long been known to inhibit neutrophil activation by chemoattractants (201, 202) and the generation of superoxide anion is one of the cellular responses most sensitive to this inhibitory pathway (27, 203). Could the phosphorylation of Rap1A mediate the inhibitory effect of cAMP on the oxidase system?

It is apparent that much additional study is required to define the role(s) of Rap1A in the oxidase system and whether other G proteins may be involved as well. At this stage, however, Rap1A is a clear frontrunner as a modulatory of guanine nucleotide regulatory effects on the NADPH oxidase system. [Our laboratory has recently succeeded in purifying a low-molecular-weight GTP binding protein from human neutrophil cytosol which exhibits stimulatory regulatory activity in the cell-free NADPH oxidase system. This protein has been identified as Rac2 (216)].

Models for Rap1A Action

At this point of little certain knowledge, it is possible to speculate about a number of potential roles for Rap1A, or another G protein, in the oxidase system. Four such possibilities, each not mutually exclusive, are discussed briefly here.

Rap1A Regulates the Binding of Cytochrome b to Other Oxidase Proteins

In this scenario Rap1A is proposed to modulate the ability of cytochrome *b* to couple effectively with other oxidase components, particularly the p47 and flavin protein, which are likely to interact directly with the cytochrome. Translocation of p47 to the plasma membrane has been shown to be defective in chronic granulomatous disease patients lacking cytochrome *b*, suggesting that it may be involved in p47 binding to the membrane (204, 205). Rap1A might regulate the conformation of the cytochrome, enabling it to effectively bind p47, or could directly mediate an interaction of the cytochrome with the p47. This activity of Rap1A could presumably be regulated by its GTP/GDP state. Similar mechanisms could be operative to regulate interaction and/or electron transfer between the cytochrome and the flavin-containing protein suggested to be a part of the oxidase system (206). Such a role for Rap1A would be consistent with the known functions of G proteins in general; namely, that they mediate the reversible interaction of macromolecules and regulate this interaction by their own state of occupation by GTP versus GDP.

Rap1A Directs Vectoral Trafficking of Cytochrome b-Containing Granules to Relevant Plasma Membrane Sites

Rap1A has been reported to be present in neutrophil granule fractions (183, 207), as is the majority of cytochrome b_{558} in resting cells (208, 209). Indeed, the two proteins appear to colocalize to the same pool of granules (199). It is possible that Rap1A could direct the specific translocation of cytochrome *b* in such vesicles to the plasma membrane, where they could become available for NADPH oxidase activity. Such a model for Rap1A action could explain its association with cytochrome b_{558} upon purification from stimulated cells, and would be consistent with the action of the Rab LMWGs to perform a similar function in the various steps of intracellular protein trafficking.

Rap1A Mediates Interaction of Oxidase Components with the Cell Cytoskeleton

This model places Rap1A in the role of an indirect modulator of the oxidase system by mediating interactions of oxidase components with cytoskeletal elements associated with the plasma membrane. A role of the membrane cytoskeleton is the regulation of oxidase in an as yet undefined fashion is indicated by a significant amount of data. Cytoskeletal interactions inhibitable by dihydrocytochalasin B may down-regulate the oxidative burst and could be involved in terminating activation by chemoattractants (210). Jesaitis and co-workers (210, 211) provided evidence for the organization of oxidase components into a plasma membrane domain associated with, and perhaps regulated by, cytoskeletal proteins. More recently, p47 was reputed to translocate to the plasma membrane via a cytoskeletal "intermediate" (212). Moreover, the *src* homology (SH3) regions found in p47 and p67 are present in several cytoskeletal binding proteins (213). Thus, the interaction with the membrane cytoskeleton may be an important means of regulating either activation or termination of the system. Several pieces of apocryphal information indicate that Rap1A could play a role in such interactions. In human platelets Rap1B was reported to become associated with the Triton X-100-insoluble cytoskeleton upon cell activation by thrombin (166). Additionally, a Rap1 homolog in the yeast *S. cerevisiae*, referred to as RSR1, has been implicated in regulating cytoskeleton-dependent processes such as budding (214).

Rap1A Is an Inhibitory Regulator of the NADPH Oxidase

This model basically suggests that Rap1A does not function in a stimulatory capacity in the NADPH oxidase system, but may serve as a means by which the system is inhibited. For example, Rap1A may occupy the normal p47 binding site on the cytochrome, preventing it from binding under "unstimulated" conditions. Some regulatory event initiated by stimuli which turn on the oxidase would cause Rap1A to dissociate from the cytochrome, freeing it for binding p47. Another scenario would envision that it is only when Rap1A is phosphorylated that it produces its inhibitory effect on the oxidase. Presumably, this inhibitory effect would be mediated at the level of the cytochrome *b*.

Variations and modifications of each of these scenarios are readily constructed at this point. Future studies in our laboratory (as well as those of other laboratories in this field, we are sure) will be directed at defining the role of Rap1A, and potentially other G proteins, in regulating components of the NADPH oxidase system.

Summary and Conclusions

The role of oligomeric G proteins in signal transduction in neutrophils has been well established, and recent work has demonstrated that they are physically coupled to their cognate receptors. With the recent cloning of these chemoattractant receptors, it should soon be possible to gain a better understanding of the specificity of receptor–G protein interactions by coexpression and reconstitution. Also, the role of pertussis toxin-insensitive G proteins can be addressed. The more recently identified LMWGs have already been implicated in the regulation of a wide variety of normal cellular processes. These include protein trafficking and processing, cytoskeletal assembly, ion fluxes, secretion, growth, and differentiation. Thus, it is perhaps no great surprise that neutrophils reflect this variety of cellular functions in their content of LMWGs. Several of these proteins may exist as remnants of cellular functions necessary during the growth and differentiation of premyeloid cells. However, it is likely that at least some of these proteins are involved in regulating the highly specialized functions of the mature phagocyte. It remains for neutrophil biologists to define these LMWGs involved in the specific functions of neutrophils which relate to their primary role as professional phagocytes. The mechanisms by which these LMWGs will act to regulate such functions as chemotaxis, aggregation, superoxide generation, and granule secretion also need to be elucidated. Additionally, we need to determine whether the LMWGs are mediators, or perhaps regulators, of the signals generated via the receptor-associated oligomeric G proteins, or whether they transduce separate novel signals. Finally, the complexities resulting from the regulation of the low-molecular-weight GTPases by extrinsic protein factors and/or lipids will require the application of novel approaches to the study of neutrophil biology.

Acknowledgments

We are grateful to Betty Goddard for secretarial assistance and to C. J. Der and M. I. Simon for providing data prior to publication. We also acknowledge J. E. Buss for contributing data for Fig. 4. Work in the authors' laboratory was supported by U.S. Public Health Service grant GM39434 to G.M.B. G.M.B. is an Established Investigator of the American Heart Association. L.A.Q. is the recipient of a research fellowship from the American Heart Association, California Affiliate, with funds contributed by the San Diego County Chapter.

References

1. E. L. Becker, *J. Leukocyte Biol.* **47,** 378–389 (1990).
2. L. Birnbaumer, J. Abramowitz, A. Yatani, K. Okabe, R. Mattera, R. Graf, J. Sanford, J. Codina, and A. M. Brown, *CRC Crit. Rev. Biochem. Mol. Biol.* **25,** 225–244 (1990).
3. C. J. Der, *in* "Oncogenes" (C. Benz and E. Liu, eds.), pp. 73–119. Kluwer Academic, Boston, Massachusetts, 1989.
4. A. Hall, *Science* **249,** 635–640 (1990).
5. M. Freissmuth, P. J. Casey, and A. G. Gilman, *FASEB J.* **3,** 2125–2131 (1989).
6. H. R. Bourne, D. A. Sanders, and F. McCormick, *Nature (London),* **348,** 125–132 (1990).
7. H. R. Bourne, D. A. Sanders, and F. McCormick, *Nature (London),* **349,** 117–127 (1991).
8. K. A. Sullivan, R. T. Miller, S. B. Masters, B. Beiderman, W. Heideman, and H. R. Bourne, *Nature (London),* **330,** 648–650 (1987).
9. R. A. Cerione, S. Kroll, R. Rajaram, C. Unson, P. Goldsmith, and A. M. Spiegel, *J. Biol. Chem.* **263,** 9345–9352 (1988).

10. H. E. Hamm, D. Deretic, M. R. Mazzoni, C. A. Moore, J. S. Takahashi, and M. M. Rasenick, *J. Biol. Chem.* **264,** 11475–11482 (1989).
11. R. Weingarten, L. Ransnas, H. Mueller, L. A. Sklar, and G. M. Bokoch, *J. Biol. Chem.* **265,** 11044–11049 (1990).
12. F. Quan, L. Thomas, and M. Forte, *Proc. Natl. Acad. Sci. U.S.A.* **88,** 1898–1902 (1991).
13. S. B. Masters, K. A. Sullivan, R. T. Miller, B. Beiderman, N. G. Lopez, J. Ramachandran, and H. R. Bourne, *Science* **241,** 448–451 (1988).
14. S. Osawa, N. Dhanasekaran, C. W. Woon, and G. L. Johnson, *Cell* **636,** 697–706 (1990).
15. S. E. Navon and B. K.-K. Fung, *J. Biol. Chem.* **262,** 15746–15751 (1987).
16. J. E. Buss, S. M. Mumby, P. J. Casey, and A. G. Gilman, *Proc. Natl. Acad. Sci. U.S.A.* **84,** 7493–7497 (1987).
17. S. M. Mumby, R. O. Heukeroth, J. I. Gordon, and A. G. Gilman, *Proc. Natl. Acad. Sci. U.S.A.* **87,** 728–732 (1990).
18. M. E. Linder, I.-H. Pang, R. J. Duronio, J. I. Gordon, P. C. Sternweis, and A. G. Gilman, *J. Biol. Chem.* **266,** 4654–4659 (1991).
19. C. J. Schmidt and E. J. Neer, *J. Biol. Chem.* **266,** 4538–4544 (1991).
20. W. F. Simonds, J. E. Butrynski, N. Gautam, C. G. Unson, and A. M. Spiegel, *J. Biol. Chem.* **266,** 5363–5366 (1991).
22. B. K.-K. Fung, *J. Biol. Chem.* **258,** 10495–10502 (1983).
23. V. A. Florio and P. C. Sternweis, *J. Biol. Chem.* **260,** 3477–3483 (1985).
24. K. J. Blumer, and J. Thorner, *Proc. Natl. Acad. Sci. U.S.A.* **87,** 4363–4367 (1990).
25. P. C. Sternweis, *J. Biol. Chem.* **261,** 631–637 (1986).
26. M. Whiteway, L. Hougan, D. Dignard, D. Y. Thomas, L. Bell, G. C. Saari, F. J. Grant, P. O'Hara, and U. L. MacKay, *Cell* **56,** 467–477 (1989).
27. R. I. Sha'afi and T. F. P. Molski, *Prog. Allergy* **42,** 1–64 (1988).
28. G. M. Bokoch, *Curr. Top. Membr. Transp.* **35,** 65–101 (1989).
29. E. A. Dennis, S. G. Rhee, M. M. Billah, and Y. A. Hannun, *FASEB J.* **5,** 2068–2077 (1991).
30. G. M. Bokoch and A. G. Gilman, *Cell* **39,** 301–308 (1984).
31. C. D. Smith, B. C. Lane, I. Kusaka, M. W. Verghese, and R. Snyderman, *J. Biol. Chem.* **260,** 5875–5878 (1985).
32. C. Koo, R. J. Lefkowitz, and R. Snyderman, *J. Clin. Invest.* **72,** 748–753 (1983).
33. L. A. Sklar, G. M. Bokoch, D. Button, and J. E. Smolen, *J. Biol. Chem.* **262,** 135–139 (1987).
34. F. Boulay, M. Tardif, L. Brouchon, and P. Vignais, *Biochem. Biophys. Res. Commun.* **168,** 1103–1109 (1990).
35. F. Boulay, M. Tardif, L. Brouchon, and P. Vignais, *Biochemistry* **29,** 11123–11133 (1990).
36. K. M. Thomas, H. Y. Pyun, and J. Navarro, *J. Biol. Chem.* **265,** 20061–20064 (1990).
37. N. P. Gerard and C. Gerard, *Nature (London)* **349,** 614–617 (1991).
38. F. Boulay, L. Mery, M. Tardif, L. Brouchon, and P. Vignais, *Biochemistry* **30,** 2993–2999 (1991).
39. Z. Honda, M. Nakamura, I. Miki, M. Minami, T. Watanabe, Y. Seyama, H. Okada, H. Toh, K. Ito, T. Miyamoto, and T. Shimizu, *Nature (London)* **349,** 342 (1990).
40. C. D. Strader and R. A. F. Dixon, *Cell. Mol. Mech. Inflamm.* **1,** 35–53 (1990).
41. G. Milligan, *Cell. Signal.* **15,** 411–419 (1989).
42. J. R. Didsbury, Y.-S. Ho, and R. Snyderman, *FEBS Lett.* **211,** 160–164 (1987).
43. J. R. Didsbury and R. Snyderman, *FEBS Lett.* **219,** 259–263 (1987).
44. G. M. Bokoch, K. Bickford, and B. P. Bohl, *J. Cell Biol.* **106,** 1927–1936 (1988).
45. P. G. Polakis, R. J. Uhing, and R. Snyderman, *J. Biol. Chem.* **263,** 4969–4976 (1988).
46. S. J. Siciliano, T. E. Rollins, and M. S. Springert, *J. Biol. Chem.* **265,** 19568–19574 (1990).
47. P. Gierschik, D. Sidirpoulos, and K. H. Jakobs, *J. Biol. Chem.* **264,** 21470–21473 (1989).

48. T. Iiri, M. Tohkin, N. Morishina, Y. Ohoki, M. Ui, and T. Katada, *J. Biol. Chem.* **264,** 21394–21400 (1989).
49. M. Tohkin, N. Morishima, T. Iiri, K. Takahashi, M. Ui, and T. Katada, *Eur. J. Biochem.* **195,** 527–533 (1991).
50. T. E. Rollins, S. Siciliano, S. Kobayashi, D. N. Cianciarulo, V. Bonilla-Argudo, K. Collier, and M. S. Springer, *Proc. Natl. Acad. Sci. U.S.A.* **88,** 971–975 (1991).
51. A. J. Jesaitis, J. O. Tolley, G. M. Bokoch, and R. A. Allen, *J. Cell Biol.* **109,** 2783–2790 (1989).
52. R. K. Bommakanti, G. M. Bokoch, D. W. Siemsen, K.-N. Klotz, J. O. Tolley, and A. J. Jesaitis, *J. Biol. Chem.* **267,** in press.
53. C. D. Smith, C. C. Cox, and R. Snyderman, *Science* **232,** 5875–5878 (1986).
54. J. C. Anthes, S. Eckel, M. I. Siegel, R. W. Egan, and M. M. Billah, *Biochem. Biophys. Res. Commun.* **163,** 657–664 (1989).
55. Y. Kanaho, H. Kanoh, and Y. Nozawa, *FEBS Lett.* **279,** 249–252 (1991).
56. G. R. Dubyak, D. S. Cowen, and L. M. Meuller, *J. Biol. Chem.* **263,** 18108–18117 (1988).
57. M. Strathmann, T. M. Wilkie, and M. I. Simon, *Proc. Natl. Acad. Sci. U.S.A.* **86,** 7407–7409 (1989).
58. M. Strathmann and M. I. Simon, *Proc. Natl. Acad. Sci. U.S.A.* **87,** 9113–9117 (1990).
59. H. K. W. Fong, K. K. Yoshimoto, P. Eversole-Cire, and M. I. Simon, *Proc. Natl. Acad. Sci. U.S.A.* **85,** 3066–3070 (1988).
60. A. V. Smrcka, J. R. Hepler, K. O. Brown, and P. C. Sternweis, *Science* **251,** 804–807 (1991).
61. T. Amatruda, D. Steele, V. Slepak, and M. I. Simon, *Proc. Natl. Acad. Sci. U.S.A.* **88,** (1991).
62. E. Santos and A. R. Nebreda, *FASEB J.* **3,** 2151–2163 (1989).
63. J. Downward, *Trends Biochem. Sci.* **15,** 469–472 (1990).
64. D. R. Kaplan, D. K. Morrison, G. Wong, F. McCormick, and L. T. Williams, *Cell* **61,** 125–133 (1990).
65. L. C. Cantley, K. R. Auger, C. Carpenter, B. Duckworth, A. Graziani, R. Kapeller, and S. Soltoff, *Cell* **64,** 281–302 (1991).
66. L. A. Quilliam, C. J. Der, and J. H. Brown, *Second Messengers Protein Phosphorylation* **13,** 59–67 (1990).
67. J. B. Gibbs, M. S. Marshall, E. M. Scolnick, R. A. F. Dixon, and U. S. Vogel, *J. Biol. Chem.* **265,** 20437–20442 (1990).
68. M. R. Smith, S. J. DeGudicibus, and D. W. Stacey, *Nature (London)* **320,** 540–543 (1986).
69. A. Yatani, K. Okabe, R. Halenbeck, P. Polakis, F. McCormick, and A. M. Brown, *Cell* **60,** 769–776 (1990).
70. T. Okamoto, T. Asano, S.-I. Harada, E. Ogata, and I. Nishimoto, *J. Biol. Chem.* **266,** 1085–1091 (1991).
71. D. G. Lowe and D. V. Goeddel, *Mol. Cell. Biol.* **7,** 2845–2856 (1987).
72. P. Chardin and A. Tavitian, *Nucleic Acids Res.* **17,** 4380 (1989).
73. V. Pizon, P. Chardin, I. Lerosey, B. Olofsson, and A. Tavitian, *Oncogene* **3,** 201–204 (1988).
74. V. Pizon, I. Lerosey, P. Chardin, and A. Tavitian, *Nucleic Acids Res.* **16,** 7719 (1988).
75. C.-A. Ohmstede, F. X. Farrell, B. R. Reep, K. J. Clemetson, and E. G. Lapetina, *Proc. Natl. Acad. Sci. U.S.A.* **87,** 6527–6531 (1990).
76. L. A. Quilliam, C. J. Der, R. Clark, E. O'Rourke, K. Zhang, F. McCormick, and G. M. Bokoch, *Mol. Cell. Biol.* **10,** 2901–2908 (1990).
77. M. T. Quinn, C. A. Parkos, L. Walker, S. H. Orkin, M. C. Dinauer, and A. J. Jesaitis, *Nature (London)* **342,** 198–200 (1989).
78. H. Kitayama, Y. Sugimoto, T. Matsuzaki, Y. Ikawa, and M. Noda, *Cell* **56,** 77–84 (1989).

79. M. Kawata, Y. Matsui, J. Kondo, T. Hishida, Y. Teranishi, and Y. Takai, *J. Biol. Chem.* **263,** 18965–18971 (1988).
80. P. Chardin, P. Madaule, and A. Tavitian, *Nucleic Acids Res.* **16,** 2717 (1988).
81. J. Didsbury, R. F. Weber, G. M. Bokoch, T. Evans, and R. Snyderman, *J. Biol. Chem.* **264,** 16378–16382 (1989).
82. K. Shinjo, J. G. Koland, M. J. Hart, V. Narasimhan, D. I. Johnson, T. Evans, and R. A. Cerione, *Proc. Natl. Acad. Sci. U.S.A.* **87,** 9853–9857 (1990).
83. S. Munemitsu, M. A. Innis, R. Clark, F. McCormick, A. Ullrich, and P. Polakis, *Mol. Cell. Biol.* **87,** 5977–5982 (1990).
84. L. A. Quilliam, J.-C. Lacal, and G. M. Bokoch, *FEBS Lett.* **247,** 221–226 (1989).
85. A. Sekine, M. Fujiwara, and S. Narumiya, *J. Biol. Chem.* **264,** 8602–8605 (1989).
86. P. Chardin, P. Boquet, P. Madaule, M. R. Popoff, E. J. Rubin, and D. M. Gill, *EMBO J.* **8,** 1087–1092 (1989).
87. H. F. Paterson, A. J. Self, M. D. Garrett, I. Just, K. Aktories, and A. Hall, *J. Cell Biol.* **111,** 1001–1007 (1990).
88. L. Reibel, O. Dorseuil, R. Stancou, J. Bertoglio, and G. Gacon, *Biochem. Biophys. Res. Commun.* **175,** 451–458 (1991).
89. H. D. Schmitt, M. Puzicha, and D. Gallwitz, *Cell* **53,** 635–647 (1988).
90. W. E. Balch, *Trends Biochem. Sci.* **15,** 473–477 (1990).
91. A. Zahraoui, N. Touchot, P. Chardin, and A. Tavitian, *J. Biol. Chem.* **264,** 12394–12401 (1989).
92. M. V. Milburn, L. Tong, A. M. DeVos, A. Brunger, Z. Yamaizumi, S. Nishimura, and S.-H. Kim, *Science* **247,** 939–945 (1990).
93. S. R. Holbrook and S.-H. Kim, *Proc. Natl. Acad. Sci. U.S.A.* **86,** 1751–1755 (1989).
94. E. F. Pai, U. Krengel, G. A. Petsko, R. S. Goody, W. Kabsch, and A. Wittinghofer, *EMBO J.* **9,** 2351–2359 (1990).
95. I. Schlichting, S. C. Almo, G. Rapp, K. Wilson, K. Petratos, A. Lentfer, A. Wittinghofer, W. Kabsch, E. F. Pai, G. A. Petsko, and R. S. Goody, *Nature (London)* **345,** 309–315 (1990).
96. M. Trahey and F. McCormick, *Science* **238,** 542–545 (1987).
97. M. D. Garrett, A. J. Self, C. van Oers, and A. Hall, *J. Biol. Chem.* **264,** 10–13 (1989).
98. A. Kikuchi, T. Sasaki, S. Araki, Y. Hata, and Y. Takai, *J. Biol. Chem.* **264,** 9133–9136 (1989).
99. P. G. Polakis, B. Rubinfeld, T. Evans, and F. McCormick, *Proc. Natl. Acad. Sci. U.S.A.* **88,** 239–243 (1991).
100. E. S. Burstein, K. Linko-Sentz, Z. Lu, and I. G. Macara, *J. Biol. Chem.* **266,** 2689–2692 (1991).
101. G. A. Martin, D. Viskochil, G. Bollag, P. C. McCabe, W. J. Crosier, H. Haubruck, L. Conroy, R. Clark, P. O'Connell, R. M. Cawthon, M. A. Innis, and F. McCormick, *Cell* **63,** 843–849 (1990).
102. C. Cales, J. F. Hancock, C. J. Marshall, and A. Hall, *Nature (London)* **332,** 548–551 (1988).
103. U. S. Vogel, R. A. F. Dixon, M. D. Schaber, R. E. Diehl, M. S. Marshall, E. M. Scolnick, I. S. Sigal, and J. B. Gibbs, *Nature (London)* **335,** 90–93 (1988).
104. F. McCormick, *Cell* **56,** 5–8 (1989).
105. I. S. Sigal, J. B. Gibbs, J. D'Alonzo, and E. M. Scolnick, *Proc. Natl. Acad. Sci. U.S.A.* **83,** 4725–4729 (1986).
106. J. C. Stone, W. C. Vass, B. M. Willumsen, and D. R. Lowy, *Mol. Cell. Biol.* **8,** 3565–3569 (1988).
107. K. Zhang, J. E. DeClue, W. C. Vass, A. G. Papageorge, F. McCormick, and D. R. Lowy, *Nature (London)* **346,** 754–756 (1990).
108. J. Downward, J. D. Graves, P. H. Warne, S. Rayter, and D. A. Cantrell, *Nature (London)* **346,** 719–723 (1990).

109. J. B. Gibbs, M. D. Schaber, T. L. Schofield, E. M. Scolnick, and I. S. Sigal, *Proc. Natl. Acad. Sci. U.S.A.* **86,** 6630–6634 (1989).
110. F. McCormick, *Nature (London)* **340,** 678–679 (1989).
111. Y. Hata, A. Kikuchi, T. Sasaki, M. D. Schaber, J. B. Gibbs, and Y. Takai, *J. Biol. Chem.* **265,** 7104–7107 (1990).
112. M. Frech, J. John, V. Pizon, P. Chardin, A. Tavitian, R. Clark, F. McCormick, and A. Wittinghofer, *Science* **249,** 169–171 (1990).
113. K. Zhang, M. Noda, W. C. Vass, A. G. Papageorge, and D. R. Lowy, *Science* **249,** 162–165 (1990).
114. P. A. Hart and C. J. Marshall, *Oncogene* **5,** 1099–1101 (1990).
115. M. J. Campa, K.-J. Chang, L. Molina y Vidia, B. R. Reep, and E. G. Lapetina, *Biochem. Biophys. Res. Commun.* **174,** 1–5 (1991).
116. A. Yatani, L. A. Quilliam, A. M. Brown, and G. M. Bokoch, *J. Biol. Chem.* **266,** 22222–22227 (1991).
117. J. Becker, T. J. Tan, H.-H. Trepte, and D. Gallwitz, *EMBO J.* **10,** 785–792 (1991).
118. H. Plutner, R. Schwaninger, S. Pind, and W. E. Balch, *EMBO J.* **9,** 2375–2383 (1990).
119. J. C. Lacal and S. A. Aaronson, *Mol. Cell. Biol.* **6,** 1002–1009 (1986).
120. S. Hattori, D. J. Clanton, T. Satoh, S. Nakamura, Y. Kaziro, M. Kawakita, and T. Y. Shih, *Mol. Cell. Biol.* **7,** 1999–2002 (1987).
121. I. Rey, P. Soubigou, L. Debussche, C. David, A. Morgat, P. E. Bost, J. F. Mayaux, and B. Tocque, *Mol. Cell. Biol.* **9,** 3904–3910 (1989).
122. B. M. Willumsen, A. G. Papageorge, H.-F. Kung, E. Bekesi, T. Robins, M. Johnsen, C. V. Vass, and D. R. Lowy, *Mol. Cell. Biol.* **6,** 2646–2654 (1986).
123. A. Wolfman and I. G. Macara, *Science* **248,** 67–69 (1990).
124. J. Downward, R. Riehl, L. Wu, and R. A. Weinberg, *Proc. Natl. Acad. Sci. U.S.A.* **87,** 5998–6002 (1990).
125. M. West, H.-F. Kung, and T. Kamata, *FEBS Lett.* **259,** 245–248 (1990).
126. D. Broek, T. Toda, T. Michaeli, L. Levin, C. Birchmeier, M. Zoller, and M. Wigler, *Cell* **48,** 789–799 (1987).
127. I. Rey, F. Schweighoffer, I. Barlat, J. Camonis, E. Boy Marcotte, R. Guilbaud, M. Jacquet, and B. Tocque, *Oncogene* **6,** 347–349 (1991).
128. T. Yamamoto, K. Kaibuchi, T. Mizuno, M. Hiroyoshi, H. Shirataki, and Y. Takai, *J. Biol. Chem.* **265,** 16626–16634 (1990).
129. T. Ueda, A. Kikuchi, N. Ohga, J. Yamamoto, and Y. Takai, *J. Biol. Chem.* **265,** 9373–9380 (1990).
130. T. Sasaki, A. Kikuchi, S. Araki, Y. Hata, M. Isomura, S. Kuroda, and Y. Takai, *J. Biol. Chem.* **265,** 2333–2337 (1990).
131. Y. Fukumoto, K. Kaibuchi, Y. Hori, H. Fujioka, S. Araki, T. Ueda, A. Kikuchi, and Y. Takai, *Oncogene* **5,** 1321–1328 (1990).
132. Y. Matsui, A. Kikuchi, S. Araki, Y. Hata, J. Kondo, Y. Teranishi, and Y. Takai, *Mol. Cell. Biol.* **10,** 4116–4122 (1990).
133. S. Kawamura, K. Kaibuchi, M. Hiroyoshi, Y. Hata, and Y. Takai, *Biochem. Biophys. Res. Commun.* **174,** 1095–1102 (1991).
134. M. Isomura, A. Kikuchi, O. Nobuyuki, and Y. Takai, *Oncogene* **6,** 119–124 (1991).
135. S. Araki, K. Kaibuchi, T. Sasaki, Y. Hata, and Y. Takai, *Mol. Cell. Biol.* **11,** 1438–1447 (1991).
136. H. R. Bourne, *Cell* **53,** 669–671 (1988).
137. M. Hiroyoshi, K. Kaibuchi, Y. Hata, and Y. Takai, *J. Biol. Chem.* **266,** 2962–2969 (1991).
138. W. A. Maltese, *FASEB J.* **4,** 3319–3328 (1990).

139. B. M. Willumsen, K. Norris, A. G. Papageorge, N. L. Hubbert, and D. R. Lowy, *EMBO J.* **3,** 2581–2585 (1984).
140. J. E. Buss, L. A. Quilliam, K. Kato, P. J. Casey, P. A. Solski, G. Wong, R. Clark, F. P. McCormick, G. M. Bokoch, and C. J. Der, *Mol. Cell. Biol.* **11,** 1523–1530 (1991).
141. J. F. Hancock, A. I. Magee, J. E. Childs, and C. J. Marshall, *Cell* **57,** 1167–1177 (1989).
142. P. J. Casey, P. A. Solski, C. J. Der, and J. E. Buss, *Proc. Natl. Acad. Sci. U.S.A.* **86,** 8323–8327 (1989).
143. J. H. Jackson, C. G. Cochrane, J. R. Bourne, P. A. Solski, J. E. Buss, and C. J. Der, *Proc. Natl. Acad. Sci. U.S.A.* **87,** 3042–3046 (1990).
144. M. Kawata, C. C. Farnsworth, Y. Yoshida, M. H. Gelb, J. A. Glomset, and Y. Takai, *Proc. Natl. Acad. Sci. U.S.A.* **87,** 8960–8964 (1990).
145. J. R. Didsbury, R. J. Uhing, and R. Snyderman, *Biochem. Biophys. Res. Commun.* **171,** 804–812 (1990).
146. H. K. Yamane, C. C. Farnsworth, H. Xie, T. Evans, W. N. Howald, M. H. Gelb, J. A. Glomset, S. Clarke, and B. K.-K. Fung, *Proc. Natl. Acad. Sci. U.S.A.* **88,** 286–290 (1991).
147. Y. Yoshida, M. Kawata, M. Katayama, H. Horiuchi, Y. Kita, and Y. Takai, *Biochem. Biophys. Res. Commun.* **175,** 720–728 (1991).
148. L. Gutierrez, A. I. Magee, C. J. Marshall, and J. F. Hancock, *EMBO J.* **8,** 1093–1098 (1989).
149. J. F. Hancock, K. Cadwallader, and C. J. Marshall, *EMBO J.* **10,** 641–646 (1991).
150. J. B. Gibbs, *Cell* **65,** 1–4 (1991).
151. P. S. Backlund, W. F. Simonds, and A. M. Spiegel, *J. Biol. Chem.* **265,** 15572–15576 (1990).
152. S. M. Mumby, P. J. Casey, A. G. Gilman, S. Gutowski, and P. C. Sternweis, *Proc. Natl. Acad. Sci. U.S.A.* **87,** 5873–5877 (1990).
153. Y. Reiss, S. J. Stradley, L. M. Gierasch, M. S. Brown, and J. L. Goldstein, *Proc. Natl. Acad. Sci. U.S.A.* **88,** 732–736 (1991).
154. R. Khosravi-Far, R. J. Lutz, A. D. Cox, L. Conroy, J. R. Bourne, M. Sinensky, W. E. Balch, J. E. Buss, and C. J. Der, *Proc. Natl. Acad. Sci. U.S.A.* **88,** 6264–6268 (1991).
155. D. A. Winegar, L. Molina y Vedia, and E. G. Lapetina, *J. Biol. Chem.* **266,** 4381–4386 (1991).
156. J. F. Hancock, H. Paterson, and C. J. Marshall, *Cell* **63,** 133–139 (1990).
157. N. Nakayama, A. Miyajima, and K. Arai, *EMBO J.* **4,** 2643–2648 (1985).
158. M. D. Resh and H.-P. Ling, *Nature (London)* **346,** 84–86 (1990).
159. M. Gatica, C. C. Allende, M. Antonelli, and J. E. Allende, *Proc. Natl. Acad. Sci. U.S.A.* **84,** 324–328 (1987).
160. P. S. Backlund and R. R. Askamit, *J. Biol. Chem.* **263,** 15864–15867 (1988).
161. H. Akbar, D. A. Winegar, and E. G. Lapetina, *J. Biol. Chem.* **266,** 4387–4391 (1991).
162. M. Kawata, A. Kikuchi, M. Hoshijima, K. Yamamoto, E. Hashimoto, H. Yamamura, and Y. Takai, *J. Biol. Chem.* **264,** 15688–15695 (1989).
163. G. M. Bokoch and L. A. Quilliam, *Biochem. J.* **267,** 407–411 (1990).
164. E. G. Lapetina, J. C. Lacal, B. R. Reep, and L. Molina y Vidia, *Proc. Natl. Acad. Sci. U.S.A.* **86,** 3131–3134 (1989).
165. L. A. Quilliam, H. Mueller, B. P. Bohl, V. Prossnitz, L. A. Sklar, C. J. Der, and G. M. Bokoch, *J. Immunol.* **147,** 1628–1635 (1991).
166. T. H. Fischer, M. N. Gatling, J.-C. Lacal, and G. C. White, *J. Biol.Chem.* **265,** 19405–19408 (1990).
167. N. Sahyoun, O. B. McDonald, F. Farrell, and E. G. Lapetina, *Proc. Natl. Acad. Sci. U.S.A.* **88,** 2643–2647 (1991).
168. Y. Hata, K. Kaibuchi, S. Kawamura, M. Hiroyoshi, H. Shirataki, and Y. Takai, *J. Biol. Chem.* **266,** 6571–6577 (1991).

169. W. Siess, D. A. Winegar, and E. G. Lapetina, *Biochem. Biophys. Res. Commun.* **170,** 944–950 (1990).
170. E. Bailly, N. Touchot, A. Zahraoui, B. Goud, and M. Bornens, *J. Cell Biol.* **111,** 343a (1990).
171. T. Yamashita, K. Yamamoto, A. Kikuchi, M. Kawata, J. Kondo, T. Hishida, Y. Teranishi, H. Shiku, and Y. Takai, *J. Biol. Chem.* **263,** 17181–17188 (1988).
172. R. Ballester, M. E. Furth, and O. M. Rosen, *J. Biol. Chem.* **262,** 2688–2695 (1987).
173. M. J. Hart, P. G. Polakis, T. Evans, and R. A. Cerione, *J. Biol. Chem.* **265,** 5990–6001 (1990).
174. G. M. Bokoch and C. A. Parkos, *FEBS Lett.* **227,** 66–70 (1988).
175. G. M. Bokoch, C. A. Parkos, and S. M. Mumby, *J. Biol. Chem.* **263,** 16744–16749 (1988).
176. E. Sarndahl, M. Lindroth, T. Bengtssen, M. Fallman, J. Gustavssen, O. Stendahl, and T. Andersson, *J. Cell. Biol.* **109,** 2791–2799 (1990).
177. T. Bengtssen, E. Sarndahl, O. Stendahl, and T. Andersson, *Proc. Natl. Acad. Sci. U.S.A.* **87,** 2921–2925 (1990).
178. G. P. Downey, C. K. Chan, and S. Grinstein, *Biochem. Biophys. Res. Commun.* **164,** 700–705 (1989).
179. S. Therrien and P.-H. Naccache, *J. Cell Biol.* **109,** 1125–1132 (1989).
180. T. Stearns, M. C. Willingham, D. Botstein, and R. A. Kahn, *Proc. Natl. Acad. Sci. U.S.A.* **87,** 1238–1242 (1990).
181. R. Weber, T. Evans, P. Polakis, R. Snyderman, and J. Didsbury, *FASEB J.* **3,** A509 (1989).
182. I. Maridonneau-Parini, C.-Z. Yang, M. Bornens, and B. Goud, *J. Clin. Invest.* **87,** 901–907 (1991).
183. M. R. Phillips, S. B. Abramson, S. L. Kolasinski, K. A. Haines, G. Weissmann, and M. G. Rosenfeld, *J. Biol. Chem.* **266,** 1289–1298 (1991).
184. M. M. Barrowman, S. Cockcroft, and B. D. Gomperts, *Nature (London)* **319,** 504–507 (1986).
185. B. D. Gomperts, *Trends Biochem. Sci.* **11,** 290–292 (1986).
186. S. Cockcroft, T. W. Howell, and B. D. Gomperts, *J. Cell Biol.* **105,** 2745–4750 (1987).
187. T. W. Howell, S. Cockcroft, and B. D. Gomperts, *J. Cell Biol.* **105,** 191–197 (1987).
188. D. Bar-Gagi and B. D. Gomperts, *Oncogene* **3,** 463–469 (1988).
189. T. G. Gabig, D. English, L. P. Akard, and M. J. Schell, *J. Biol. Chem.* **262,** 1685–1690 (1987).
190. R. Seifert, W. Rosenthal, and G. Schultz, *FEBS Lett.* **205,** 161–164 (1986).
191. J. Doussiere, M.-C. Pilloud, and P. V. Vignais, *Biochem. Biophys. Res. Commun.* **152,** 993–1001 (1988).
192. P. E. Nasmith, G. B. Mills, and S. Grinstein, *Biochem. J.* **257,** 893–897 (1989).
193. P. Peveri and J. T. Curnutte, *Blood,* **74,** 397a (1989).
194. R. A. Clark, *J. Infect. Dis.* **161,** 1140–1147 (1990).
195. E. Ligeti, J. Doussiere, and P. V. Vignais, *Biochemistry* **27,** 193–200 (1988).
196. B. G. J. M. Bolscher, S. W. Denis, A. J. Verhoeven, and D. Roos, *J. Biol. Chem.* **265,** 15782–15787 (1990).
197. H. Nunoi, D. Rotrosen, J. I. Gallin, and H. L. Malech, *Science* **242,** 1298–1301 (1988).
198. T. G. Gabig, E. A. Eklund, G. B. Potter, and J. R. Dykes, *J. Immunol.* **145,** 945–951 (1990).
199. A. J. Jesaitis, L. McPhail, R. A. Clark, G. M. Bokoch, and M. T. Quinn, *FASEB J.* **4,** A2179 (1990).
200. G. M. Bokoch, L. A. Quilliam, B. P. Bohl, A. J. Jesaitis, and M. T. Quinn, *Science,* **254,** 1794–1796 (1991).
201. H. Mueller, H. J. Motulsky, and L. A. Sklar, *Mol. Pharmacol.* **34,** 347–353 (1988).
202. H. Mueller and L. A. Sklar, *J. Cell. Biochem.* **40,** 27–34 (1989).
203. I. Rivkin, J. Rosenblatt, and E. L. Becker, *J. Immunol.* **115,** 1126–1134 (1975).
204. D. Rotrosen and T. L. Leto, *J. Biol. Chem.* **265,** 19910–19915 (1990).
205. P. G. Heyworth, J. T. Curnutte, W. M. Nauseef, B. D. Volpp, D. W. Pearson, H. Rosen, and R. A. Clark, *J. Clin. Invest.* **87,** 352–356 (1991).

206. C. M. Yea, A. R. Cross, and O. T. G. Jones, *Biochem. J.* **265,** 95–100 (1990).
207. M. T. Quinn, M. Mullen, and J. Linner, *J. Cell. Biochem., Suppl.* **15C,** 202 (1991).
208. N. Borregard, J. M. Heiple, E. R. Simons, and R. A. Clark, *J. Cell Biol.* **97,** 52–60 (1983).
209. A. J. Jesaitis, E. S. Buescher, D. Harrison, M. T. Quinn, C. A. Parkos, S. Livesy, and J. Linner, *J. Clin. Invest.* **85,** 821–835 (1990).
210. A. J. Jesaitis and R. A. Allen, *J. Bioenerg. Biomembr.* **20,** 679–707 (1988).
211. M. T. Quinn, C. A. Parkos, and A. J. Jesaitis, *Biochim. Biophys. Acta* **987,** 83–94 (1989).
212. W. M. Nauseef, B. D. Volpp, S. McCormick, K. G. Leidal, and R. A. Clark, *J. Biol. Chem.* **266,** 5911–5917 (1991).
213. D. G. Drubin, J. Mulholland, Z. Zhu, and D. Botstein, *Nature (London)* **343,** 288–290 (1990).
214. A. Bender and J. R. Pringle, *Proc. Natl. Acad. Sci. U.S.A.* **86,** 9976–9980 (1989).
215. G. M. Bokoch and U. Prossnitz, *J. Clin. Invest.* **89,** in press (1992).
216. U. G. Knaus, P. G. Heyworth, T. Evans, J. T. Curnutte, and G. M. Bokoch, *Science* **254,** 1512–1515 (1991).

CHAPTER 3

Regulation of Phospholipase C Isozymes

Sue Goo Rhee, Do Joon Park, and Dongeun Park

Laboratory of Biochemistry
National Heart, Lung, and Blood Institute
National Institutes of Health
Bethesda, Maryland 20892

In response to the binding of various ligands to their cell surface receptors, it is well documented that phosphoinositide (PI)-specific phospholipase C (PLC) catalyzes the hydrolysis of phosphatidylinositol 4,5-bisphosphate (PIP_2) and generates two second messenger molecules, inositol 1,4,5-trisphosphate (IP_3) and diacylglycerol. The transmembrane signaling events that underlie the coupling of receptor occupancy to PLC activation is, however, not clearly understood. Evidence accumulated over the past several years suggests that there are multiple forms of PLC in eukaryotic cells and that there are several distinct mechanisms by which the various PLC isoforms are activated. The stimulation of specific receptors appears to result in the activation of specific PLC isozymes.

Activation of PLC by G Protein-Dependent and -Independent Pathways

The results of numerous studies have implicated a mediatory, and mandatory, role of GTP-binding proteins in transduction of the signal from

Cellular and Molecular Mechanisms of Inflammation, Volume 3

receptor to PLC. Therefore, by analogy with the well-characterized receptor-linked adenylate cyclase and retinal cGMP phosphodiesterase systems, heterotrimeric G proteins have been suggested to play the role of transducer. However, several studies have also suggested that receptor signals can be transduced to PLC independently of G proteins.

On the basis of their predicted amino acid sequences, most receptors can easily be categorized into one of a few superfamilies, such as growth factor receptors and G protein-coupled receptors. Receptors for platelet-derived growth factor (PDGF), epidermal growth factor (EGF), and fibroblast growth factor (FGF) differ from other hormone receptors that stimulate PI hydrolysis in that they possess intrinsic tyrosine-specific protein kinase activity (1, 2). Furthermore, these growth factor receptors share little or no amino acid sequence similarity or predicted structural similarity with the superfamily of G protein-coupled receptors (3). The mode of PLC activation initiated by PDGF and EGF appears to be different from that initiated by G protein-coupled receptors (3–9). The observed differences include the absence or presence of a lag period between receptor stimulation and PIP_2 hydrolysis, the effects of prior treatment of cells with phorbol 12-myristate 13-acetate (PMA), and, most importantly, GTP or GTP analogs.

PDGF, vasopressin, and bombesin are potent mitogens for Swiss 3T3 cells, the rat fibroblast cell line WFB, and various other cells. Binding of these mitogens to cell surface receptors elicits the hydrolysis of PIP_2, which leads to rapid intracellular responses that include an increase in cytosolic free Ca^{2+} concentration ($[Ca^{2+}]_i$) and activation of protein kinase C (PKC). On stimulation of WFB cells by PDGF, there is a lag period of approximately 10 sec before an increase in $[Ca^{2+}]_i$ is observed, but no measurable lag period is observed for the Ca^{2+} response induced by vasopressin or bombesin (5). Pretreatment of WFB cells with PMA profoundly inhibits inositol phosphate formation evoked by vasopressin and bombesin, but enhances to some extent inositol phosphate formation induced by PDGF (5). In membranes prepared from WFB cells or in WFB cells made permeable to nucleotides, GTP or the nonhydrolyzable analog GTPγS markedly enhances the vasopressin- and bombesin-stimulated PI hydrolysis, but has no effect on PDGF-stimulated PI hydrolysis (5). Similar experiments with permeabilized Swiss 3T3 cells (4) have indicated that GTPγS potentiates the coupling of bombesin receptors to PLC, whereas the activation of PLC by PDGF occurs in a manner that is unaffected by GTPγS.

In an extensive study with rat liver epithelial WB cells, Hepler *et al.* (8) provided evidence that the EGF receptor and receptors for adrenaline, angiotensin II, and [Arg⁸]vasopressin stimulate PIP_2 hydrolysis by independent pathways. The time courses for accumulation of inositol phosphates in response to angiotensin II and EGF were markedly different.

Whereas angiotensin II stimulated a rapid accumulation of inositol phosphates (maximal by 30 sec), increases in the levels of inositol phosphates in response to EGF were measurable only after a 30-sec lag period; maximal levels were attained after 7–8 min. Under experimental conditions in which agonist-induced desensitization no longer occurred in these cells, the inositol phosphate responses to EGF and angiotensin II were additive, whereas those to angiotensin II and [Arg^8]vasopressin were not. In crude WB cell lysates, angiotensin II, [Arg^8]vasopressin, and adrenaline each stimulated inositol phosphate formation in a guanine nucleotide-dependent manner. In contrast, EGF failed to stimulate inositol phosphate formation in WB cell lysates in the presence or absence of GTPγS, even though EGF retained the capacity to bind to and stimulate tyrosine phosphorylation of its receptor.

The results obtained with WFB cells (5), Swiss 3T3 cells (4), and WB cells (8) thus demonstrate that receptors for bombesin, adrenaline, angiotensin II, and [Arg^8]vasopressin are apparently coupled to activation of PLC by G proteins. In contrast, G proteins do not appear to contribute to the actions of EGF and PDGF receptors in these cells.

It should be noted, however, that EGF-stimulated inositol phosphate accumulation in rat hepatocytes was shown to be abolished by pertussis toxin treatment (7), suggesting the possible involvement of a G protein in EGF receptor action in rat liver. Furthermore, in permeabilized vascular smooth muscle cells, the ability of PDGF to stimulate inositol phosphate formation was found to be synergistically increased by the presence of GTPγS, although pertussis toxin did not inhibit PDGF-dependent PLC activation (9). Therefore, it is possible that the mechanisms by which the growth factor receptors stimulate PLC and the sensitivity of these mechanisms to pertussis toxin might vary in different cell types.

Heterogeneity in the PI Response to Specific Ligands

The PI response to a specific ligand varies between tissues and cell types, a finding that has been partly attributed to the molecular diversity of receptors. Recently, molecular cloning and expression of individual members of receptor families have accelerated our understanding of the roles of receptors in mediating the responses to ligands in target cells. For example, cDNAs and genes for five different muscarinic acetylcholine receptors (m_1–m_5) have been cloned (10–12). The individual expression of different cloned receptors in the same host cell has allowed the responses of the receptors to be examined in a controlled environment, and it has become clear that differences in responses are due to the receptors. The m_1, m_3, and m_5 receptors transfected into mammalian cells have been shown to stimulate PI hydrolysis and cAMP accumulation through a pertussis toxin-insensitive G protein (13–16). These three receptor subtypes belong to the M_1 pharmacological type, which is characterized by a high affinity for pirenzepine, and are structurally more related to each other than they are to the M_2 type, which includes the m_2 and m_4 receptors. The M_2 receptors have low affinity for pirenzepine and are associated with inhibition of adenylate cyclase (13, 17). The role of M_2 type receptors in PI signaling is not clear. There are indications that the m_2 and m_4 receptors, when expressed at high levels in CHO and embryonic kidney cells, can couple weakly to PI stimulation through pertussis toxin-sensitive G protein at high doses of agonist (13, 17). However, expression and stimulation of m_2 and m_4 receptors in NG108 and A9L cells have been shown to have no detectable stimulatory effect on PI hydrolysis (15, 16). Furthermore, in rat thyroid FRTL5 cells, which contain an M_2 muscarinic receptor, the cholinergic agonist carbachol decreases both basal and adrenergic receptor-dependent PI turnover (18). These results demonstrate that M_2 receptors of the same type may be coupled to different second messenger systems in different cells and tissues.

Cell type-dependent coupling to second messenger systems has also been observed with dopamine receptors. There are two main types of dopamine receptors (D_1 and D_2) identified and several novel subtypes of both D_1 and D_2 receptors have been identified (19). Stimulation of D_1 receptors causes activation of adenylyl cyclase and often stimulates PI turnover (19). The D_2 receptors are widely regarded as typical inhibitory receptors because they inhibit both adenylyl cyclase and PI turnover (19). The mechanism of this latter effect is somewhat controversial: some studies have shown the PI inhibition to be secondary to an effect on K^+ channel activation (20), whereas others have suggested a direct inhibitory effect on PLC (21). The D_2 receptor has been cloned and expressed in two different cell lines, pituitary GH_4C_1 cells and LtK^- fibroblasts. The D_2 receptor induced inhibition of adenylyl cyclase in both cells, but different responses of PI turnover despite the similar levels of receptor expression. In GH_4C_1 cells, D_2 receptors failed to affect PI hydrolysis, whereas in LtK^- cells the D_2 receptors induced rapid stimulation of inositol phosphate formation. Therefore, as with muscarinic M_2 receptors, the PI response to the D_2 receptor appears to depend on the cell type on which the receptor is expressed.

The simplest explanation for such heterogeneous responses is that the postreceptor components—G proteins and PLC—required for PI signaling are differentially expressed in different cells. It is noteworthy that at least two types of G proteins, pertussis toxin-sensitive and -insensitive forms, participate in PI signaling and that, as discussed in the next section, a number of PLC isoforms exist in mammalian tissues.

Multiple Forms of PLC

PI-specific phospholipase C (PLC) is present in most mammalian cells, as well as in plants and various microorganisms (22–24). A number of distinct PLC enzymes have been purified from a variety of mammalian tissues (22), and several forms have been molecularly cloned and sequenced (25–30). Comparison of their deduced amino acid sequences and immunological cross-reactivity indicates that mammalian PLCs can be divided into three types—PLC-β, PLC-γ, and PLC-δ—each of which is a discrete gene product (22). All three forms of PLC are single-polypeptide enzymes, with molecular masses measured by SDS–PAGE of 150–154 kDa for PLC-β (31–34), 145–148 kDa for PLC-γ (31–33), and 85–88 kDa for PLC-δ (31–33).

All three enzymes have similar catalytic properties: they hydrolyze the three common phosphoinositides, PI, PI-4P, and PI-4,5-P_2, but not PI-3P, PI-3,4-P_2, or PI-3,4,5-P_3 (35, 36); and their catalytic activities are dependent on the concentration of Ca^{2+}. Nevertheless, a noticeable difference is apparent in the capacities of these three enzymes to generate cyclic inositol phosphates. Hydrolysis of PI, PI-4-P, and PI-4,5-P_2 by PLC enzymes yields cyclic and noncyclic inositol phosphates (37). The ratio of cyclic to noncyclic products was shown to decrease in the order PLC-β > PLC-δ > PLC-γ, when the hydrolysis of PI, PI-4-P, and PI-4,5-P_2 was measured under different pH and Ca^{2+} concentrations (38). For example, the average value of 1,2-cyclic, 4,5-trisphosphate produced by PLC-β, PLC-δ, and PLC-γ was 5.3, 3.7, and 0.6%, respectively, at pH 7.0 and a Ca^{2+} concentration below 500 μM. Recently. Majerus and colleagues (39) demonstrated that cells with lower levels of cyclic inositol phosphates grow to a lower density at confluence, suggesting that cyclic inositol phosphates play a role in the control of cell proliferation. Thus, it is likely that activation of different PLC isoforms can exert different effects on the long-term cell growth, even when the initial concentrations of IP_3 and diacylglycerol generated by the PLC enzymes are identical.

The PLC isoforms appear to respond differently to changes in the intracellular level of cAMP (40). Evidence suggests that activation of cAMP-dependent protein kinase (PKA) attenuates receptor-coupled PLC activity, thus providing a mechanism for cross-talk between the PI signaling and cAMP signaling cascades. The possible targets of PKA action appear to include PLC-γ (40). Thus, in cells containing PLC-β, PLC-γ, and PLC-δ, PKA has been shown to selectively phosphorylate PLC-γ (40).

The three types of PLC enzymes are dissimilar not only in molecular size but also in amino acid sequence. This lack of sequence similarity is consistent with the absence of immunological cross-reactivity between the three enzymes. When the sequences of PLC-β, PLC-γ, and PLC-δ originally isolated from rat and bovine brains are compared, despite a low overall homology between the three enzymes, a significant sequence similarity is apparent in two domains, one of about 150 amino acids and the other of about 240 amino acids (41). The two domains, designated X and Y in Fig. 1, are about 60 and 40% identical, respectively, between the three PLCs [the extent of the Y domain is greater than previously recognized (22)]. The two X and Y domains might constitute, separately or jointly, an important region responsible for catalytic properties, such as the specific recognition of Ca^{2+} and phosphoinositides or the hydrolysis of the phosphodiester bond. Each of the three enzymes contains an amino terminal 300 amino acid region which precedes the X domain. Sequence similarity in this region is only 20%.

Bacterial PI-specific PLC recognizes the inositol phosphate structure present in PI, but does not hydrolyze the more highly phosphorylated

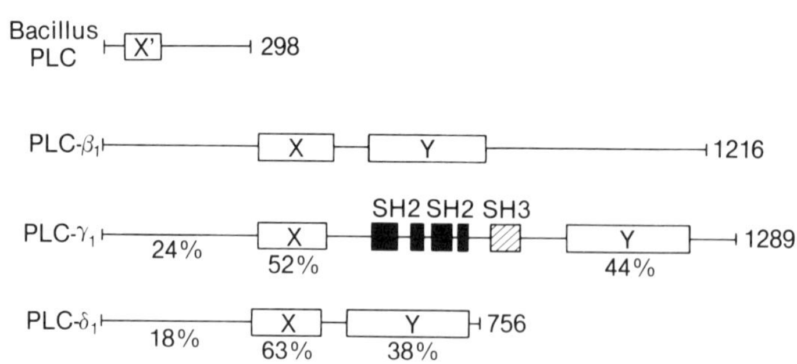

FIGURE 1

Linear display of *Bacillus* PLC and three types of mammalian PLCs (β, γ, and δ types) represented by PLC-β_1, PLC-γ_1, and PLC-δ_1. Open boxes X and Y denote the regions of approximately 150 and 240 amino acids, respectively, of similar sequence found in the three types of mammalian PLC. Part of the X region is conserved in *Bacillus* PLC and is designated X′. The numbers at the right of the representations are the numbers of amino acid residues in each molecule. The percentage values under the various domains of PLC-γ_1 and PLC-δ_1 refer to the percentage identity with the corresponding domains in PLC-β_1.

derivatives of PI, PI-4P, and PI-4,5-P_2 (24). The bacterial enzymes also catalyzes the hydrolysis of the glycosyl-PI-anchor, thereby converting membrane-bound proteins to soluble forms. Bacterial PLC does not require divalent cations for activity. The genes for PLC from *Bacillus thuringiensis* (23) and *Bacillus cereus* (24) have been cloned and sequenced. Amino acid sequences of the two *Bacillus* enzymes are nearly identical, and at 298 amino acids, *Bacillus* PLCs are much smaller than the mammalian enzymes. Yet a relatively high degree of similarity (20% identity; 40% similarity including conservative replacements) between the *Bacillus* enzymes and mammalian brain PLC is apparent in a 70-amino acid segment located in the X domain (24). This observation further supports the hypothesis that active sites of PLCs might reside in the conserved domain of X. The smaller X domain found in *Bacillus* PLC is referred to as the X′ domain in Fig. 1.

When we began to use Greek letters to designate the PLC isozymes, we assigned PLC-α to the 62–68 kDa enzymes purified initially from rat liver and sheep seminal vesicles and later from guinea pig uterus (22). These 62–68 kDa enzymes appeared to be immunologically distinct from PLC-β, PLC-γ, and PLC-δ, and the amino acid sequence deduced from a putative PLC-α cDNA showed no similarity to those of the other PLC enzymes. The PLC-α cDNA was obtained from rat basophilic leukemic cell libraries with the use of rabbit serum raised against the 62 kDa guinea pig uterus PLC (29). The protein encoded by this putative PLC-α clone showed most similarity to thioredoxin and protein disulfide isomerase. No sequence corresponding to the X and Y domains could be located in the deduced sequence of PLC-α. Furthermore, because the PLC-α cDNA has not been expressed, whereas the cDNAs for *Bacillus* PLC, PLC-β, PLC-γ, and PLC-δ have been expressed to demonstrate a concomitant increase in PLC activity, the question of whether the rat basophilic leukemia cell cDNA actually encodes a PLC has been raised. Recently, Martin *et al.* (42) convincingly showed that the rat basophilic leukemia cell cDNA actually encodes an endoplasmic reticulum protein that carries no PLC activity.

In an attempt to find additional types of PLC, cDNAs from various tissues have been screened by low stringency cross-hybridization with probes based on the conserved domain X or Y. As a result, four new PLC-related cDNAs have been cloned and sequenced (30, 41, 43). Sequence alignment of the four new PLCs with the three brain PLCs revealed that each of the new sequences is similar to and is structurally related to one of the three previously isolated PLCs. This result suggests that each PLC type (β, γ, and δ) contains several distinct members. Greek letters have thus been used to designate the types of PLC with different primary structures and arabic subscript numerals to designate the members of each type. The original three enzymes isolated from mammalian brain are named PLC-β_1, PLC-γ_1, and PLC-δ_1. The difference in primary structures of different members of a PLC type is not due to differences in the species or tissues of origin. For example, amino acid conservation is better than 95% for PLC-γ_1 from rat, bovine, and human brains and PLC-γ_1 can be found in almost every mammalian tissue.

One of the new cDNA clones, isolated from a HL-60 library, encodes an enzyme most closely related to PLC-β_1 and is referred to as PLC-β_2. The *Drosophila* PLC gene (44), *NorpA*, most closely resembles the PLC-β type. The PLC-β type has a carboxyl-terminal 400-amino acid domain that contains an unusually high number of charged residues (about 40%) in this region. Another feature of the PLC-β type is the presence of a string of nearly consecutive acidic residues in the region between the X and Y domains; the *NorpA* enzymes, however, does not possess this acidic domain. The PLC-δ type of isozyme is readily distinguishable by the lack of a carboxy-terminal region after the Y domain. PLC-δ_2 has been purified to homogeneity from bovine brain and PLC-δ_3 cDNA has been isolated from a WI-38 fibroblast library.

PLC-γ_2 cDNA have been obtained from libraries of human lymphocytes (45), rat muscle (30), and HL-60 cells (43) by low-stringency hybridization techniques. PLC-γ_1 and PLC-γ_2 have high sequence identities in the amino-terminal 300 amino acids and in the 400-amino acid region between the X and Y domains. In the 400-amino acid insert between X and Y, PLC-γ_1 and PLC-γ_2 contain three regions that are related in sequence to limited portions of the *src* product (25, 26). The three regions correspond to duplicates of SH_2 and to SH_3 (*src* homology 2 and 3), which were first recognized as highly conserved sequences in the regulatory domains of a number of nonreceptor tyrosine kinases, such as those encoded by *abl, yes, fgr, lyn, syn, hck, lck,* and *blk* (the catalytic region of these *src*-related tyrosine kinases is named SH_1) (46).

PLC-γ isozymes can, therefore, be structurally divided into three domains, X, Y, and SH (SH_2 plus SH_3). In order to study the function of each domain, various plasmids encoding truncated PLC-γs were constructed and expressed either in *Escherichia coli* (PLC-γ_2) (30) or transiently in COS-1 cells (PLC-γ_1) (47). PLC activity was clearly detected when the SH domain was deleted, although the activity was reduced to 10–30% of full-length enzyme. However, deletion in either the X or Y domain led to a complete loss of activity. It appears, therefore, that X and Y, but not SH, are essential for PLC activity.

Another interesting sequence similarity was noticed by Baker (48) between a 100-residue segment of the carboxy terminal half of PLC-γ and the constant region 2 (C_2 domain) of PKC. There are 31% identities and 16%

conservative replacements. Extending this observation, we found that the carboxy-terminal half of the Y domain in all three types of PLC (β, γ, and δ) is similar to the C_2 domain of PKC. The PKC C_2 domain is present in all PKC isoforms that translocate to membranes in response to submicromolar concentrations of Ca^{2+}, but is absent in PKC isoforms that fail to translocate in response to Ca^{2+}. The C_2 domain is therefore believed to be important for the Ca^{2+}-dependent binding of PKC to membranes. Recently, Clark *et al.* (49) noticed that a region homologous to the PKC C_2 domain also exists in the amino-terminal portion of an 85 kDa phospholipase A_2 (PLA_2). PLA_2 is in the cytosol of unstimulated cells but translocates to the membrane in response to increased concentrations of Ca^{2+}. Furthermore, a 16 kDa amino-terminal fragment of PLA_2 that contains the C_2-like domain associates with membrane vesicles in a Ca^{2+}-dependent manner. These results led Clark *et al.* to suggest that the C_2-like sequence of PLA_2 encodes a Ca^{2+}-dependent phospholipid-binding domain. It is therefore reasonable to speculate that the C_2-like sequence located in the Y domain of all mammalian PLCs also serves as a Ca^{2+}-dependent phospholipid-binding motif. This speculation is consistent with the fact that mammalian PLCs require Ca^{2+} for catalytic activity, whereas the activity of the *Bacillus* enzymes, which lack the Y domain, is independent of Ca^{2+}.

All of the PLC enzymes described above are presumed to be located within cells. Extracellular PI-specific PLC has been found at the external cell surface of Swiss 3T3 cells with the use of a fluorescent analog of PI (50). This enzyme was dependent on Ca^{2+} for activity. The level of this extracellular enzyme increased after 3T3 cells became confluent, suggesting that this PLC may play a role in the density-dependent inhibition of cell growth. Whether this extracellular PLC represents another new type of enzyme is not known.

G Protein-Dependent Activation of PLC

The members of the G protein family mediate the coupling of many cell surface receptors to various signal transduction mechanisms. There are more than 13 members in the G protein family (51–53), all of which are heterotrimers composed of α, β, and γ subunits. The α subunits, which contain the guanine nucleotide binding site, show the greatest sequence diversity and generally define the different G proteins. An agonist-occupied receptor activates G proteins by catalyzing the exchange of bound GDP for GTP. Binding of GTP leads to the dissociation of the βγ subunit complex from the α-GTP. The α-GTP complex as well as βγ subunit are known to regulate the activity of specific enzymes and ion channels. The β and γ subunits of different G proteins are highly homologous and, at least *in vitro,* are functionally interchangeable so that they may associate with any of the different α subunits.

The best-defined transmembrane signaling system, which has been studied for many years, is the adenylyl cyclase system where the roles of stimulatory G protein (G_s) and inhibitory G protein (G_i) have been well characterized (51). Evidence also indicates that G proteins participate not only in the activation, but also in the inhibition, of PLC activity. By analogy with the nomenclature used for the adenylyl cyclase system, putative G proteins that stimulate and inhibit PLC have been called $G_{p(s)}$ and $G_{p(i)}$, respectively.

A role for G proteins in coupling receptor activation to PIP_2 breakdown was first suggested from the results of studies on the effects of guanine nucleotide on the binding of various Ca^{2+}-mobilizing agonists to their receptors. The presence of GTP decreased the binding affinity of agonists such as angiotensin II, vasopressin, α_1-adrenergic agonist, *f* Met–Leu–Phe, thyrotropin-releasing hormone (TRH), and muscarinic agonists (54, 55). In analogy with the adenylyl cyclase system, this observation was interpreted as an indication for the involvement of G proteins (G_p). According to the model for the coupling of adenylyl cyclase to G_s, the interaction of agonist with the receptor leads to the formation of a high-affinity receptor–agonist-G_s complex which, upon interaction with GTP, dissociates to α_s-GTP, βγ, and low-affinity agonist-receptor complexes.

The most direct evidence for the involvement of a G protein in receptor regulation of PLC comes from studies with cell-free preparations where GTP (or GTP analogs) has been shown to cause the breakdown of PIP_2 in the absence of agonist or to potentiate the receptor-mediated PLC activation. Cockcroft and Gomperts (56) showed that GTPγS and other non-hydrolyzable GTP analogs stimulate the breakdown of polyphosphoinositide in plasma membrane preparations from human neutrophils. Similarly, GTPγS-dependent hydrolysis of phosphoinositide has been observed with rat liver plasma membranes (57) and turkey erythrocyte membranes (58). Litosch *et al.* (59) also reported that GTP was required for agonist-induced breakdown of polyphosphoinositide in cell-free extracts of fly salivary glands.

Fluoride, in the millimolar concentration range, is a general activator of G proteins, probably because AlF_4^-, formed from F^- and Al^{3+}, mimics the γ phosphate of GTP, thereby converting GDP-bound, inactive G proteins to an activated form. In a number of cell types, addition of NaF, often together with $AlCl_3$, to prelabeled cells or isolated membranes has been shown to stimulate the formation of inositol phosphates.

The bacterial toxin, pertussis toxin, provided further evidence favoring the involvement of G proteins in PLC activation. ADP-ribosyltransferase, a subunit of the toxin, penetrates cells and uses endogenous NAD to ADP ribosylate a cysteine near the carboxy terminus of the G protein α subunits, α_i, α_t, and α_o (60, 61). The α_s, which lacks a cysteine residue in this position, is not a substrate for pertussis toxin. ADP-ribosylation by pertussis toxin appears to cause uncoupling of G proteins from receptors (60), which results in inhibition of agonist-activated pathways regulated by the G proteins.

In many cells, agonist-triggered PI breakdown is inhibited by pertussis toxin, whereas in others transduction is unaffected by the toxin. This indicates that there are at least two distinct $G_{p(s)}$ proteins. It appears that a single cell can express both pertussis toxin-sensitive and -insensitive $G_{p(s)}$ proteins. Thus, in human umbilical vein endothelial cells, pertussis toxin blocks stimulation of PI turnover by histamine but does not affect PI turnover stimulated by bradykinin (62). Similar results have been obtained with cultured rat sensory neurons, where neuropeptide Y and bradykinin both elevate inositol phosphate formation (63). The neuropeptide Y-stimulated inositol phosphate formation is blocked by treatment with pertussis toxin; whereas the effects of bradykinin are unaltered by the toxin, despite the fact that the bradykinin-dependent PI turnover is mediated by a G protein as indicated by the synergistic effects of bradykinin and GTPγS on this process (63).

In order to investigate whether a single cell can possess multiple $G_{p(s)}$ proteins and whether distinct $G_{p(s)}$ proteins can couple selectively to different receptors, Ashkenazi *et al.* (64) expressed three subtypes of muscarinic receptors—m_1, m_2, and m_3—in CHO cells, which lack endogenous muscarinic receptors, and investigated the pathway employed by each muscarinic receptor, as well as that used by endogenous cholecystokinin and thrombin receptors, to activate PI hydrolysis in these cells. Carbachol evoked a significantly lower accumulation of inositol phosphates in cells expressing the m_2 receptor compared to those in cells expressing the m_1 or m_3 receptor. The level of inositol phosphate accumulation stimulated by cholecystokinin was comparable to the m_1 receptor- and m_3 receptor-mediated carbachol response, whereas the accumulation by thrombin was similar in magnitude to the m_2-mediated carbachol response. Treatment of CHO cells with pertussis toxin caused no effect on cholecystokinin-stimulated PI hydrolysis, partially inhibited (20–50%) PI hydrolysis stimulated by m_1 and m_3 receptors, and completely inhibited PI hydrolysis stimulated by m_2 and thrombin receptors. These results further indicate that at least two $G_{p(s)}$ proteins, pertussis toxin-sensitive and -insensitive $G_{p(s)}$ proteins, mediate the selective coupling of these different receptors to PI hydrolysis.

The partial inhibitory effect observed for m_1 and m_3 receptors is consistent with each receptor being coupled to both pertussis toxin-sensitive and -insensitive $G_{p(s)}$ proteins or, alternatively, with coupling of these receptors to a third $G_{p(s)}$ protein, the activity of which is only partially attenuated by the toxin.

The existence of distinct types of $G_{p(s)}$ proteins in CHO cells and their selective coupling to different receptors was further demonstrated by the additive or nonadditive nature of the PI hydrolysis responses activated by different receptors. In cells expressing m_2 receptors, the cholecystokinin and carbachol responses were fully additive, whereas the thrombin and carbachol responses were not additive. On the other hand, in cells expressing m_1 receptors, neither the cholecystokinin nor the thrombin response was additive with the carbachol response, indicating that m_1 receptors can couple to both the $G_{p(s)}$ pathways employed by cholecystokinin and thrombin (and m_2) receptors. Thus, Ashkenazi *et al.* (64) concluded that CHO cells possess a pertussis toxin-insensitive $G_{p(s)}$, which couples endogenous cholecystokinin receptors and transfected m_1 receptors to PI hydrolysis, and a pertussis toxin-sensitive $G_{p(s)}$, which couples endogenous thrombin receptors and transfected m_2 receptors, as well as transfected m_1 receptors, to PI hydrolysis.

Ashkenazi *et al.* (64) also noted that the specificity observed in the coupling of the various receptors to PI hydrolysis is similar to that observed for the same receptors in other cell types. Thus, thrombin receptors in platelets and fibroblasts, like those in CHO cells, activate PI hydrolysis via a pertussis toxin-sensitive $G_{p(s)}$. In addition, in 1321 N human astrocytoma cells and rat pancreatic islet cells, in which the primary muscarinic receptor is the m_3 subtype, carbachol-stimulated PI hydrolysis is insensitive to pertussis toxin, consistent with the primarily pertussis toxin-insensitive coupling of the m_3 receptor in CHO cells.

In contrast, Moriarty *et al.* (65) found that receptors that use the pertussis toxin-sensitive pathway in one cell type can use the pertussis toxin-insensitive $G_{p(s)}$ in other cell types. For example, the [Arg^8]vasopressin receptor, which stimulates PLC in a pertussis toxin-insensitive manner in liver, stimulates PLC through a pertussis toxin-sensitive pathway in *Xenopus* oocytes.

In addition to the heterotrimeric G protein family, there is a family of monomeric, lower molecular mass (20–30 kDa) G proteins. Lapetina and Reep (66) detected four low molecular mass G proteins of 21, 27, 29, and 29.5 kDa in platelets. The 27- and 29-kDa proteins were susceptible to degradation by trypsin, whereas the other two proteins were resistant to trypsin degradation. Since both the binding of GTP to platelet membrane proteins and the GTPγS-dependent stimulation of PLC activity were not altered by trypsin, Lapetina and Reep suggested that the two trypsin-resistant proteins might regulate PLC in platelets. McAtee and Dawson (67) proposed a 24 kDa G protein as transducer in bradykinin-induced PLC activation in NCB-20 cells. Their proposal was based on the observations that bradykinin-induced PLC activation in NCB-20 cells was inhibited by raising the cellular cAMP levels (i.e., by activating PKA) and that the phosphorylation state of the 24 kDa G protein correlated with the extent of PLC inhibition. Nevertheless, current evidence favoring a role for monomeric G proteins in PLC activation is indirect and circumstantial.

Furthermore, there is evidence to suggest that $G_{p(s)}$ proteins are trimeric. Because βγ subunits appear to attenuate α subunit-mediated stimulation of effectors in all signal transducing systems involving heterotrimeric G proteins, elevation of intracellular concentration of βγ would be expected to reduce PLC activity if $G_{p(s)}$ proteins are also heterotrimeric G proteins. To determine whether βγ subunits have such an effect, Moriarty *et al.* (65, 68) microinjected βγ subunits purified from human erythrocytes and bovine brain into *Xenopus* oocytes, in which IP_3 has been shown to mobilize intracellular Ca^{2+} and to evoke a Ca^{2+}-dependent Cl^- current. Microinjection of βγ subunits inhibited Cl^- current stimulated by carbachol, vasopressin, and cholecystokinin, suggesting that both the pertussis toxin-sensitive and -insensitive pathways for receptor coupling to PLC are transduced by heterotrimeric G proteins.

In another study with βγ subunit, Boyer *et al.* (69) used turkey erythrocyte membranes which had been known to possess a PLC that is markedly activated by P_{2y}-"purinergic" receptor agonist and GTPγS. Reconstitution of turkey erythrocyte membranes with βγ subunits resulted in inhibition of both AlF_4^--stimulated adenylate cyclase and AlF_4^--stimulated PLC activities. The apparent potency of βγ subunits for inhibition of each enzyme activity was similar, and inhibition occurred with βγ purified from turkey erythrocytes, bovine brain, or human placenta membranes. These results suggest the involvement of a G protein possessing an αβγ heterotrimeric structure in the coupling of hormone receptors to PLC.

To identify $G_{p(s)}$ proteins, Moriarty *et al.* (70) again made use of *Xenopus* oocytes, in which muscarinic receptors couple to PLC through a pertussis toxin-sensitive G protein, and measured the IP_3-sensitive Cl^- current after the microinjection of several pertussis toxin-sensitive G proteins (G_0, G_{i1}, and G_{i3}) purified from bovine brain and human erythrocytes. When the α subunits activated by GTPγS were injected, α_0 evoked a rapid Cl^- current, whereas the three activated α_i subunits (α_{i1}, α_{i2}, and α_{i3}) had no effect.

Injection of trimeric G_0 specifically enhanced the muscarinic receptor-stimulated Cl^- current. These data suggest that G_0 or a G_0-like G protein may represent a pertussis toxin-sensitive $G_{p(s)}$.

Some progress has been made in identifying the $G_{p(s)}$-coupled PLC in GH_3 cells (71) and rabbit brain (72). TRH-dependent PI turnover has been shown to be insensitive to pertussis toxin in GH_3 cells. With the use of exogenous substrate, Martin and Kowalchyk (71) found that the $G_{p(s)}$-regulated PLC in GH_3 cells is an extrinsic membrane protein and can be solubilized reversibly at high ionic strength. Cytosolic PLCs from GH_3 cells failed to substituted for the KCl-solubilized GH_3 membrane PLC in reconstituting GTPγS-stimulated PLC activity in membranes. Similarly, cytosolic PLCs from rat brain failed to reconstitute whereas the KCl-extracted brain membrane PLC could substitute for the GH_3 membrane enzyme. As such, the $G_{p(s)}$-coupled PLC in GH_3 cells is similar to brain PLC-β_1, which was reported by Lee *et al.* (73) and by Katan *et al.* (34) to be solubilized by 2 *M* KCl. In agreement with this observation, Carter *et al.* (72) found that prior incubation of brain cortical membranes with antibodies to PLC-β_1 inhibited GTPγS-stimulated PLC activity.

Despite the numerous descriptions of $G_{p(s)}$ in a variety of cell types, it was only recently that direct molecular characterizations of $G_{p(s)}$ have been achieved. Several laboratories have independently made significant contributions to identifying the long-sought pertussis toxin-insensitive $G_{p(s)}$. With the polymerase chain reaction technique, Strathman and Simon (52) obtained and sequenced cDNA clones encoding two murine Gα subunits, α_q and α_{11}, that are 88% identical. Both $G\alpha_q$ and $G\alpha_{11}$ are widely distributed and lack the cysteine residue four amino acids from the carboxyl terminal end that is the target for pertussis toxin-mediated ADP ribosylation. Pang and Sternweis (74) purified $G\alpha_q$ from rat brain with the use of an affinity matrix containing immobilized βγ subunits. This purified 42 kDa protein was not recognized by antibodies to known Gα proteins, and amino acid sequences obtained from tryptic fragments are homologous to, yet different from, those of other Gα subunits. The partial amino acid sequences were present in the sequence predicted from the α_q cDNA. The amino acid sequence information indicated that the α_q preparation also contained a second highly similar Gα subunit (α_{11}) as a minor component. Both α_q and α_{11} subunits were shown not to be substrates for ADP-ribosylation catalyzed by pertussis toxin; and they bound GTPγS only with slow rates and low stoichiometry, probably due to their high-affinity association with GDP.

Sternweis and co-workers (75) showed that the α_q preparation obtained by affinity chromatography could stimulate the activity of partially purified PLC from bovine brain, but only in the presence of AlF_4^-; no significant stimulation of activity was observed with GTPγS, which is anticipated by the inability of α_q to bind the nucleotide. The affinity of AlF_4^--activated α_q for PLC appeared to be low (K_d > 20 n*M*). Stimulation of PLC by α_q was observed over a large range of Ca^{2+} concentrations. In addition to increasing the maximal activity of PLC, α_q changed the apparent affinity of the enzyme for Ca^{2+} from ~1 to 0.1 μ*M*. Thus, PLC activation was achieved by increasing both the intrinsic activity of the enzyme and its sensitivity to the concentration of free Ca^{2+}. Maximal fold activation was observed at lower concentrations of Ca^{2+}, a finding that is consistent with observations with diverse membrane systems.

Progress in identifying a pertussis toxin-insensitive $G_{p(s)}$ has been made by Taylor *et al.* (76), who recognized that cholate-solubilized extracts of liver membranes possessed both PLC and a $G_{p(s)}$ protein, as pretreatment of membranes with GTPγS enhanced PLC activity in the cholate extracts. The GTPγS-dependent activator, $G_{p(s)}$, was purified on the basis of its ability to activate partially purified membrane PLC. Persistent impurities that copurified with the activator during several column chromatography steps included α_{i1}, α_{i2}, and α_{i3}. Therefore, the final purification step involved an incubation with pertussis toxin in the presence of NAD^+, which caused the ADP-ribosylation of α_i subunits but had been shown to exert no effect on the function of the liver activator. The $\alpha_{p(s)}$ thus separated from ADP-ribosylated α_i subunits exhibited a molecular mass of 42 kDa on SDS-polyacrylamide gel and copurified with a substoichiometric amount of β subunit. This 42 kDa $\alpha_{p(s)}$ revealed cross-reactivity with antipeptide antibodies raised against residues 160–169 of α_{i1} and a region of sequence common to all known G protein α subunits. The 42 kDa protein was not recognized by other α subunit-specific antibodies. These findings identify the purified 42 kDa activator as a distinct pertussis toxin-insensitive G protein α subunit.

In spite of the biochemical advances which have resulted in the characterization of one or two $G_{p(s)}$ proteins and multiple isoforms of PLC, it remains unclear which of the PLC isoforms is regulated by G proteins. Immunological studies have indicated that the 42 kDa $\alpha_{p(s)}$ contains α_q- plus an α_q-like protein, that is likely to be α_{11}. When the two α subunits were resolved, both had PLC stimulatory activity. Taylor *et al.* (77) reconstituted the 42 kDa α_q and the β_1, γ_1, and δ_1 isozymes of PLC purified from bovine brain. This Gα subunit specifically activated PLC-β_1, but not PLC-γ_1 and PLC-δ_1. In contrast to the observations made with α_q purified with the βγ-affinity column, the stimulation of PLC-β_1 by bovine liver membrane α_q did not result in a decreased Ca^{2+} requirement for PLC; at all free Ca^{2+} concentrations (0.02–20 μ*M*) the stimulation of PLC-β_1 was similar.

The PLC isozyme specificity of α_q was further investigated by incubating bovine liver membranes with antibodies to the various PLC isozymes. Antibodies to the β_1 isozyme inhibited the stimulatory effect of α_q by approximately 80%, while antibodies to PLC-γ_1 or PLC-δ_1 gave no inhibition. This result suggests that the main, if not the sole, target of α_q is PLC-β_1 in liver membranes.

Avian homologs of mammalian PLC-β_1 and G_q have been purified by Harden and co-workers, who have been studying the P_{2y}-purinergic receptor- and G protein-regulated PI metabolism in turkey erythrocyte membranes (78). A 150 kDa PLC has been purified from turkey erythrocytes. This PLC appears to be closely related to PLC-β_1, although it does not cross-react with antibodies raised against the latter, and, when reconstituted with PIP_2-containing phospholipid vesicles prepared from turkey erythrocyte membranes, the purified protein showed AlF_4^-- or GTPγS-stimulated PLC activity. With reconstitution of AlF_4^--sensitive PLC activity as an assay, the putative G protein conferring regulation to the 150 kDa PLC was purified (79). Two polypeptides of 43 and 35 kDa were obtained. The 43 kDa protein strongly reacted with antiserum to the carboxy terminus of α_q and α_{11}, and the 35 kDa protein was recognized by G protein β subunit antiserum. Furthermore, G protein $\beta\gamma$ subunits were shown to inhibit PLC activity stimulated by the 43 kDa protein and AlF_4^-.

G Protein-Dependent Inhibition of PLC

Evidence is gradually accumulating that PLC may also be regulated by inhibitory receptors and G proteins. Activation of certain receptors for dopamine, muscarinic agonists, adenosine, and acidic amino acids has been shown to inhibit the PI metabolism and accumulation of Ca^{2+} within cells. Two different mechanisms may be involved in these responses. Many instances of receptor-mediated inhibition of PI breakdown can be detected only after a period of several minutes and may be secondary to receptor-mediated events that lower intracellular Ca^{2+} or increase cAMP. In other instances, the activation of an inhibitory G protein, $G_{p(i)}$. The receptors that inhibit PI breakdown and their signaling pathways have been reviewed in (80); here, we will summarize several reports published since then.

D_2 dopamine receptors inhibit adenylyl cyclase in certain cell types but do not affect its activity in other cells. In addition, D_2 receptors are known to inhibit PI turnover, activate K^+ channels, and inhibit voltage-gated Ca^{2+} channels (19). Activation of D_2 receptors in pituitary lactotroph cells inhibits PI turnover induced by TRH. This inhibition was sensitive to pertussis toxin and remained unchanged by increased cellular cAMP levels but was greatly affected by treatments that modify the cytosolic free Ca^{2+} concentration. The inhibitory effect of dopamine was prevented by treatment of the cells with the Ca^{2+} ionophore ionomycin and was mimicked either by withdrawal of Ca^{2+} from the incubation medium or by blockage of voltage-gated Ca^{2+} channels with verapamil. In isolated membranes, dopamine was unable to counteract the inositol phosphate accumulation triggered by TRH. Vallar *et al.* (20) thus concluded that inhibition of PI turnover is not a primary event triggered by D_2 receptor activation, but is a consequence of the inhibition of dopamine of the prolonged increase in free Ca^{2+} concentration that is induced by TRH via activation of voltage-gated Ca^{2+} channels.

On the other hand, there is evidence suggesting the direct involvement of G proteins in the inhibition of PLC. Delahunty *et al.* (81) showed that adenosine inhibited basal and TRH-stimulated PI turnover in GH_3 cells through a mechanism which appeared to be insensitive to the removal of Ca^{2+} from the medium. Recently, Litosch (82) demonstrated that guanine nucleotides mediate both stimulatory and inhibitory effects on PLC activity of rat cerebral cortical membranes. Nonhydrolyzable GTP analogs, GTPγS and GPP(NH)P, inhibited basal PLC activity by 30% at 10 n*M*. Increasing the concentration of GTPγS or GPP(NH)P to over 10 n*M* resulted in a reversal of the inhibitory effect and onset of stimulation of PLC activity. Expression of the dual effects of guanine nucleotides was affected by the Mg^{2+} concentration. At 0.3 m*M* Mg^{2+}, both the inhibitory and the stimulatory components of GPP(NH)P action were evident, whereas at 2.5 m*M* Mg^{2+}, only stimulation was observed. These results can be best explained by the hypothesis that PLC in cerebral cortical membrane is modulated by two distinct G proteins, inhibitory $G_{p(i)}$ and stimulatory $G_{p(s)}$, and that $G_{p(i)}$ has a greater affinity for Mg^{2+} and guanine nucleotides than does $G_{p(s)}$. Similar Mg^{2+} effect was observed with adenylyl cyclase system in platelet membranes: GTPγS below 1 μ*M* inhibited adenylyl cyclase in the presence of 2 m*M* Mg^{2+}, whereas in the presence of 12 m*M* Mg^{2+}, GTPγS, at concentrations greater than 0.1 μ*M* activated adenylyl cyclase. This Mg^{2+} effect appeared to reflect higher affinities of Mg^{2+} and guanine nucleotide to G_i than to G_s.

Dose-dependent biphasic responses of inositol phosphate formation to GTPγS or AlF_4^- have also been observed in intact and permeabilized human umbilical vein endothelial cells (83). In this system, however, stimulation rather than inhibition of PLC activity was found at lower GTPγS (or AlF_4^-) concentrations. Because the biphasic responses were still present in permeabilized cells, and even in cell homogenates, it is unlikely that changes in pH, Ca^{2+} concentration, or cAMP concentration were responsible. Furthermore, elevation of intracellular cAMP by forskolin did not affect inositol phosphate levels in the presence of stimulatory or inhibitory concentrations of AlF_4^-. This demonstration of cAMP-independent modulation of PLC activity was important because in a variety of cells and tissues elevated cAMP levels have been shown to inhibit PI turnover (40).

Bizzari *et al.* (18) reported that muscarinic agonist carbachol reduced the basal levels of IP_3 and inhibited adrenergic receptor-stimulated inositol phosphate accumulation in FRTL5 rat thyroid cells. Both the adrenergic and muscarinic receptors are coupled to G proteins that are sensitive to pertussis toxin, as was made evident by the observation that both the stimulatory as well as the inhibitory pathways are inactivated by toxin treatment. However, the sensitivities of the two pathways to the toxin are very different, indicating that distinct G proteins are involved. Both the stimulatory and inhibitory pathways require the presence of GTP. Bizzari *et al.* (18) proposed that the $G_{p(i)}$ protein coupled to PLC regulation in these cells acts directly on the enzyme. This proposal was based on the following observations: (i) carbachol and GTP could induce the PLC inhibition in permeabilized cells, i.e., under the condition of extreme dilution of any soluble cellular factor; (ii) high concentration of intracellular Ca^{2+} induced by a specific ionophore in intact cells or fixed Ca^{2+} concentrations in permeabilized cells did not affect the muscarinic inhibition; (iii) carbachol was still able to decrease the PLC activity in the presence of saturating levels of cAMP in permeabilized cells, and in the presence of forskolin in intact cells; and (iv) PKC does not seem to play a role in the muscarinic inhibition because its direct activator, PMA, and the kinase inhibitor staurosporine did not interfere with the carbachol effect.

As described above, experimental data from several laboratories strongly suggest the existence of an inhibitory G protein, $G_{p(i)}$. At present, one can only speculate about the molecular mechanism of action of $G_{p(i)}$. There is no evidence to favor a role of the $\alpha_{p(i)}$ subunit versus the $\beta\gamma$ subunits in this process.

Activation of PLC by Growth Factor Receptor Tyrosine Kinases

Polypeptide growth factors such as PDGF, EGF, FGF, colony-stimulating factor (CSF-1), and insulin mediate their pleiotropic actions by binding to and activating cell surface receptors that possess intrinsic protein-tyrosine kinase (PTK) activity. These growth factor receptor tyrosine kinases have a similar molecular topology. All possess a large glycosylated, extracellular ligand-binding domain, a single hydrophobic transmembrane region, and a cytoplasmic region that contains a tyrosine kinase domain (2). Shared structural features and homologous primary structures reveal the existence of four subclasses of receptors within the receptor tyrosine kinases (2): subclass I contains the EGF receptor and the erbB-2 product; subclass II, the insulin receptor; subclass III, the PDGF and CSF-1 recep tors; and subclass IV, the FGF receptor.

Despite the structural similarities between their receptors, the role of polypeptide growth factors in PI signaling does not appear to be uniform. Binding of PDGF (5) and EGF (84, 85) to their respective receptors induce stimulation of PI turnover. In contrast, CSF-1, whose receptor is highly homologous to and has been assigned to the same subclass as the PDGF receptor, has no effect on PI turnover in mononuclear phagocytes (86). There is no consensus regarding a role for PI turnover or Ca^{2+} mobilization in the mechanisms of action of FGF. Magnaldo *et al.* (87) concluded that neither the acidic nor basic FGF receptor signaling pathway is coupled to the activation of PLC, whereas Kaibuch *et al.* (88) have presented evidence that basic FGF can rapidly induce diacylglycerol formation and Ca^{2+} mobilization. Similar discrepancies exist regarding the effect of insulin on PI metabolism. Farese *et al.* (89) showed a transient increase in the IP_3 levels in response to insulin in fat cells. However, other investigators have demonstrated in several cell lines and tissues that insulin does not generate IP_3 as a second messenger (90–92).

Recently, the mechanism by which EGF and PDGF stimulate PLC activity has been studied extensively in several laboratories. The growth factor-induced stimulation of PLC appears to be independent of G proteins (4–9) and requires the intrinsic tyrosine kinase activity of the receptors. Mutant PDGF and EGF receptors that lack tyrosine kinase activity bind the corresponding growth factor but fail to stimulate the hydrolysis of PIP_2 (93–95). Wahl *et al.* (96) found that stimulation of PLC activity by EGF in A431 cells is correlated with the retention of increased amounts of PLC activity by an immunoaffinity matrix constructed with antibodies to phosphotyrosine, suggesting that PLC, or a tightly associated protein, is a direct tyrosine phosphorylation substrate of the EGF receptor. Subsequently, Wahl *et al.* (97, 98), Meisenhelder *et al.* (99), Margolis *et al.* (100), and Kumjian *et al.* (101) showed that treatment of a number of cells with EGF or PDGF led to an increase in the phosphorylation of PLC-γ_1, but not of PLC-β_1 or PLC-δ_1. The increased phosphorylation occurred on both serine and tyrosine residues. Tyrosine phosphorylation of PLC-γ_1 occurred rapidly, reached a peak level at 0.5–2 min of growth factor treatment, and was well correlated with stimulation of PIP_2 hydrolysis (102). Growth factor internalization was not necessary for PLC-γ_1 phosphorylation on tyrosine (97, 99).

Treatment of cells with EGF or PDGF also promoted the association of PLC-γ_1 with their receptors. Thus, antibodies to either PLC-γ_1 or growth factor receptors immunoprecipitated both proteins (97–102). Both tyrosine phosphorylation of PLC-γ_1 and coimmunoprecipitation of PLC-γ_1 and receptors were reversibly lost with acid dissociation of growth factors from their receptors and recovered with the readdition of growth factor (97, 99, 101, 103). Dissociation of bound growth factor by an acid wash caused a rapid dephosphorylation of growth factor receptor and PLC-γ_1. However, if the PDGF-induced receptor phosphorylation was maintained by adding a tyrosine phosphatase inhibitor orthovanadate, the PDGF receptor could still be coprecipitated with PLC-γ_1 and still stimulate PI turnover (103). Mutant PDGF and EGF receptors (95, 104) with defective kinase activity fail to associate with PLC-γ_1. Oligomerization of the EGF receptor is not sufficient to induce association of the receptor with PLC-γ_1, since the kinase-negative mutant receptor that has been shown to undergo normal dimerization in response to EGF does not associate with PLC-γ_1 (95). The requirement of receptor autophosphorylation for association with PLC-γ_1 was further demonstrated *in vitro* by the observations that PDGF receptor expressed with recombinant baculovirus vector also associated with PLC-γ_1 and that phosphatase treatment of the baculovirus-expressed PDGF receptor greatly decreased its association with PLC-γ_1 (104).

Although the insulin receptor possesses intrinsic PTK activity, treatment of NIH 3T3 cells with mitogenic concentrations of insulin did not cause phosphorylation of PLC-γ_1 (99, 105). Neither purified intact insulin receptor nor the β-chain kinase domain was able to phosphorylate PLC-γ_1 *in vitro* (105). Similarly, although the PDGF and CSF-1 receptors are structurally related, CSF-1 treatment neither stimulated phosphorylation of PLC-γ_1 nor mobilized intracellular Ca^{2+} (106).

Tyrosine phosphorylation of PLC-γ_1 *in vitro* by purified EGF or PDGF receptors is highly specific; whereas PLC-γ_1 is an efficient substrate, PLC-β_1 is a poor substrate and PLC-δ_1 is not phosphorylated to any detectable extent (99, 107). The major sites of phosphorylation by EGF and PDGF receptors *in vivo* and *in vitro* appear to be identical (99, 104) and are tyrosine residues 472, 771, 783, and 1254. The rate of phosphorylation *in vitro* was most rapid at site 771 and 783, was slower at site 1254, and was slowest at site 472 (108).

The role of tyrosine phosphorylation was investigated by substituting phenylalanine for tyrosine at these three sites of PLC-γ_1 and expressing the mutant enzymes in NIH 3T3 cells (109). Phenylalanine substitution at tyrosine 783 completely blocked the activation of PLC by PDGF, whereas mutation at tyrosine 1254 inhibited the response by 40% and mutation at tyrosine 771 enhanced the response by 50%. The decreased response to PDGF of the cells harboring mutant PLC-γ_1 was not because the phenylalanine substitution at the tyrosines inactivated the enzymes. Mutation at residues 771, 783, or 1254 did not affect the catalytic activity of PLC-$\gamma_1$measured *in vitro.* Like the wild-type enzyme, PLC-γ_1 substituted with phenylalanine at tyrosine 783 became associated with the PDGF receptor and underwent phosphorylation at serine residues in response to PDGF. These results suggest that PLC-γ_1 is the isozyme of PLC that mediates PDGF-induced inositol phospholipid hydrolysis and that phosphorylation on tyrosine 783 is essential for PLC-γ_1 activation. Furthermore, they show that neither the association of PLC-γ_1 with the PDGF receptor nor its phosphorylation on serine residues is sufficient to account for PDGF-induced activation of PLC-γ_1. At the present time, the significance of serine phosphorylation is not known.

Molecular events which might occur during the activation of PLC-γ_1 by a growth factor receptor PTK have recently been proposed in detail (41). The proposed events include a tight interaction between the SH_2 domain of PLC-γ_1 and phosphotyrosine residues in the intracellular domain of the autophosphorylated receptor, followed by the phosphorylation of PLC-$\gamma_1$tyrosine residues 771, 783, and 1254 by the receptor kinase. Tyrosine phosphorylation may induce a major conformational change in PLC-γ_1 and allow the SH_3 domain of PLC-γ_1 to interact with membrane cytoskeleton, causing the translocation of PLC-γ_1 from the cytosol to the cellular membrane.

PLC-γ_2 also contains SH_2 and SH_3 domains and is known to be phosphorylated at unidentified tyrosine residues in response to PDGF treatment (110). In addition, whereas residues equivalent to tyrosine residues 771 and 783 of PLC-γ_1 are conserved in PLC-γ_2, an equivalent of Tyr 1254 is not present in PLC-γ_2. Therefore, one can speculate that the mechanism of activation of PLC-γ_2 also involves tyrosine phosphorylation and that PLC-γ_1 and PLC-γ_2 respond differently to a PTK and a regulatory mechanism.

Activation of PLC-γ_1 Through Tyrosine Phosphorylation by Nonreceptor PTK

Proper ligation of a variety of cell surface receptors in leukocytes results in the activation of nonreceptor PTKs and of PLC. Several laboratories have investigated the role of nonreceptor PTKs in the activation of PLC by the membrane IgM (mIgM) in B lymphocytes, the T cell antigen receptor

(TCR), the high-affinity IgE receptor ($Fc_\varepsilon RI$) in basophilic leukemia cells, and IgG receptors (FcγRs) in monocytic cells. The structures of these leukocyte receptors are shown in Fig. 2.

B cells bind antigen via mIgM molecules, which differ from secreted antibody molecules in the heavy (H) chain carboxy terminus. The H chain of mIgM contains spacer, transmembrane, and cytoplasmic sequences that are not found in secreted H chains. Each mIgM H chain has a single transmembrane-spanning region with a cytoplasmic tail consisting of only three amino acids, lysine-valine-lysine. In view of this limited cytoplasmic structure, it seems likely that mIgM transduces signals via associated proteins. Indeed, recently a disulfide-linked heterodimer of the products of *b29* and *mb1* was found to be associated with mIgM (111).

Among the early intracellular events triggered by ligation of the mIgM complex is the activation of PLC and PTKs. To determine whether these are elements of a common signal transduction pathway, Carter *et al.* (112) assessed the effect of three PTK inhibitors on mIgM signal transduction in human B-lymphoblastoid cell lines. Tyrphostin completely suppressed the increase in $[Ca^{2+}]_i$ and the generation of inositol phosphates induced by ligation of mIgM. Herbimycin and genistein reduced by 30 and 50%, respectively, the rise in $[Ca^{2+}]_i$ caused by optimal ligation of mIgM, and they abolished it in cells activated by suboptimal ligation of mIgM. These investigators also assayed immunoprecipitates obtained with anti-phosphotyrosine Ab from detergent lysates of B-lymphoblastoid cells for PLC activity. Ligation of mIgM increased immunoprecipitable PLC activity by 2-fold in 90 sec and 4-fold in 30 min. Specific immunoprecipitation and Western blot analysis identified tyrosine phosphorylation of PLC-γ_1 after 60 sec of stimulation. Thus, Carter *et al.* concluded that activation of PLC in B cells by mIgM requires PTK functions and is associated with tyrosine phosphorylation of PLC-γ_1. Candidates for the PTK include the *hck* and *lyn* products and that of a B cell-specific member of the *src* family, *blk.*

The TCR complex functions to recognize antigen and to transduce signals across the plasma membrane. The TCR complex is composed of an antigen-binding, disulfide-linked heterodimer of α and β chains that is associated with three nonpolymorphic polypeptides, γ, δ, and ε (collectively termed CD3), and with a disulfide-linked homodimer or heterodimer of ξ and η chains. Although none of the components of the TCR complex is a protein kinase, the ligation of the TCR complex activates PTK activity. Candidates for the TCR-regulated PTK include the products of *fyn* and *lck,* which are members of the *src* family. The TCR was recently shown to coimmunoprecipitate with Fyn from T cells (113) and Lck is known to be associated with the cytoplasmic tail of CD4, which functions as a coreceptor with TCR (114).

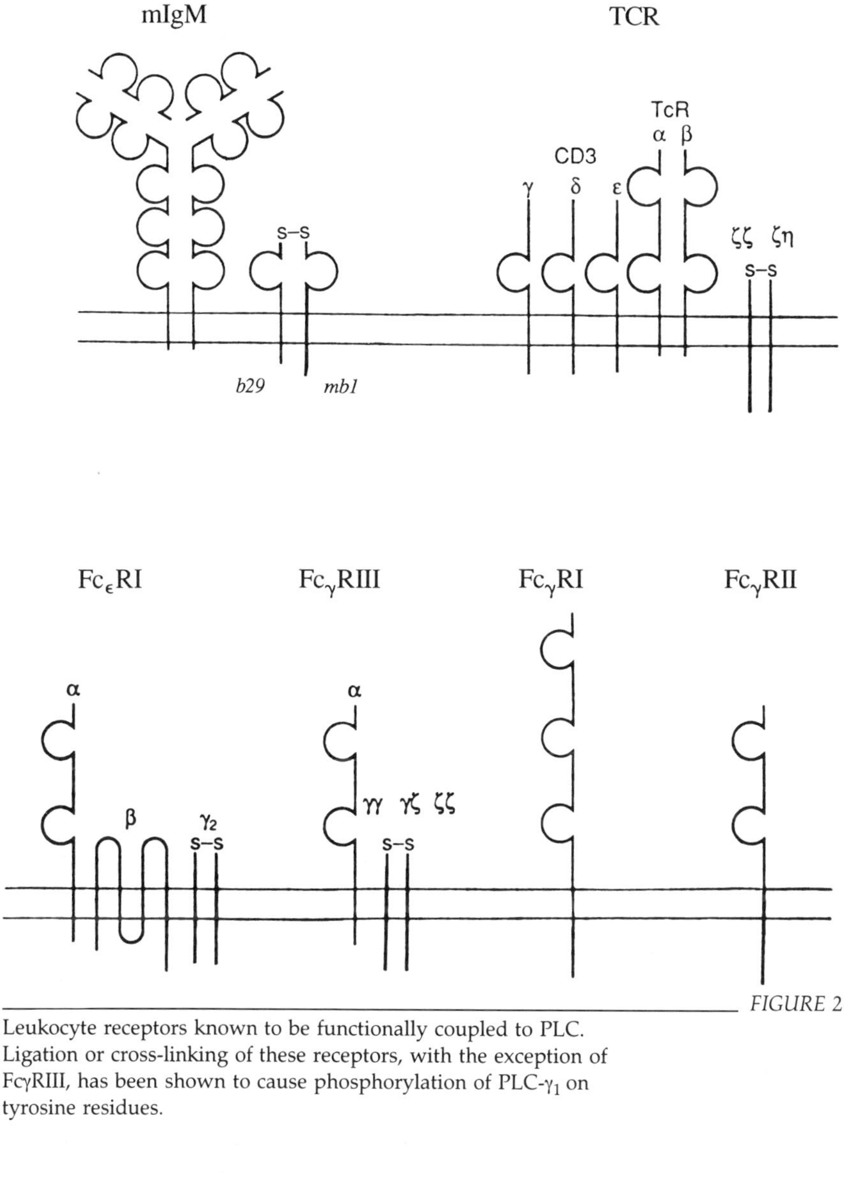

FIGURE 2

Leukocyte receptors known to be functionally coupled to PLC. Ligation or cross-linking of these receptors, with the exception of FcγRIII, has been shown to cause phosphorylation of PLC-γ_1 on tyrosine residues.

The ligation of TCR provokes a rapid increase in PLC activity. Earlier reports suggested that the TCR might belong to the large family of G protein-coupled receptors. Direct stimulation of G proteins with AlF_4^- or GTPγS was shown to activate PLC in intact or permeabilized T cell populations. Recent evidence suggests, however, that protein tyrosine phosphorylation participates in the regulatory linkage between the TCR and PLC in T cells. June *et al.* (115) demonstrated that the tyrosine phosphorylation of several intracellular proteins preceded the onset of PIP_2 hydrolysis or $[Ca^{2+}]_i$ increases in anti-CD3 antibody-stimulated T-cells. The hypothesis that protein tyrosine phosphorylation generates a positive signal for PIP_2 hydrolysis received further support from studies indicating that pharmacological inhibitors of TCR-stimulated PTK activity also block TCR-dependent PLC activation in T cells (116, 117).

Several laboratories (118–120) therefore investigated whether any of the PLC isozymes become phosphorylated in T cells in response to TCR stimulation. Park *et al.* (118) showed that the human T cell line Jurkat contains PLC-β_1 and PLC-γ_1. Treatment of Jurkat cells with antibody to CD3 led to phosphorylation of PLC-γ_1 but not of PLC-β_1. The phosphorylation of PLC-γ_1 occurred rapidly and transiently on both serine and tyrosine residues. Tyrosine phosphorylation reached a maximum level less than 1 min after stimulation and then decreased rapidly. Two-dimensional phosphopeptide map analysis revealed that the major sites of tyrosine and serine phosphorylation in PLC-γ_1 from activated Jurkat cells are the same as those in PLC-γ_1 phosphorylated in cells treated with peptide growth factors such as PDGF and EGF. Thus, this result suggests that PIP_2 hydrolysis triggered by the TCR is due, at least in part, to activation of PLC-γ_1 and that the mechanism by which this activation is achieved involves phosphorylation of multiple tyrosine residues on PLC-γ_1 by a nonreceptor tyrosine kinase coupled to the TCR complex.

$Fc_\varepsilon RI$ receptor is found exclusively on mast cells and basophils. When multivalent allergens bind to the receptor-bound IgE, the consequent aggregation of the receptors leads to the release of mediators responsible for allergic symptoms. $Fc_\varepsilon RI$ is a tetrameric complex comprised of an IgE binding α subunit, one β subunit, and a dimer of disulfide-linked γ subunits (121). The PLC-mediated hydrolysis of PIP_2 is one of the early events that follow $Fc_\varepsilon RI$ aggregation.

The molecular mechanism that couples $Fc_\varepsilon RI$ aggregation to PLC activation has been the subject of intensive study. Considerable evidence suggests that a G protein participates in the IgE-dependent activation of PLC (122, 123). Thus, GTPγS mimics the effect of IgE on secretion when introduced into the cytoplasm of mast cells and enhances the formation of inositol phosphates when added to permeabilized mast cells. This proposed role for a G protein is in harmony with the fact that $Fc_{\varepsilon}RI$ is predicted to have a total of seven transmembrane domains, as is the case for most receptors that interact with G proteins. However, the G protein hypothesis is complicated by observations showing that the responses of mast cells and cognate cells to different stimuli are not affected in the same way by pertussis toxin. The hydrolysis of PIP_2 and secretion induced by chemical stimuli, such as compound 48/80 and 5′-(*N*-ethyl)carboxamidoadenosine (NECA), are inhibited by pertussis toxin; in contrast, IgE-stimulated hydrolysis of PIP_2 is resistant to the effects of this toxin (122). These results suggest that $Fc_{\varepsilon}RI$ activates PLC through a pertussis toxin-insensitive G protein, whereas the receptors for compound 48/80 and NECA interact with a pertussis toxin-sensitive G protein. Alternatively, $Fc_{\varepsilon}RI$ may activate PLC by a G protein-independent mechanism. Indeed, Saito *et al.* (123) showed that the IgE-dependent formation of inositol phosphates in permeabilized cells was neither enhanced by GTPγS nor inhibited by GDPβS, as would be expected if a G protein was involved.

Park *et al.* (124) recently observed that the rat basophilic leukemia cell line RBL-2H3 contains PLC-γ_1, but not PLC-β_1 and PLC-δ_1, and that stimulation of these cells with oligomeric IgE elicits a rapid and transient phosphorylation of PLC-γ_1 on tyrosine residues. Prior incubation of RBL-2H3 cells with the PTK inhibitor herbimycin A prevented the tyrosine phosphorylation of PLC-γ_1, as well as the hydrolysis of PIP_2, induced by oligomeric IgE. However, NECA, which is known to activate PLC through a G protein, did not elicit tyrosine phosphorylation of PLC-γ_1. These results indicate that phosphorylation of PLC-γ_1 by a nonreceptor tyrosine kinase is the mechanism by which IgE receptor aggregation triggers PLC activation. The activation of the tyrosine kinase coupled to the IgE receptor also appears to require an active tyrosine phosphatase, because IgE-induced PLC-γ_1 tyrosine phosphorylation was prevented by phenylarsine oxide, an inhibitor of protein–tyrosine phosphatase activity.

Cross-linking of receptors for the Fc domain of IgG (FcγRs) on macrophages, monocytes, neutrophils, and natural killer (NK) cells by immune complexes or opsonized antigen activates a multitude of biological functions, such as antibody-dependent cellular cytotoxicity, phagocytosis, release of inflammatory mediators, and superoxide production (125). Three distinct classes of human FcγRs—FcγRI, FcγRII, and FcγRIII—can be distinguished on hematopoietic cells on the basis of their structures and ligand binding affinities (125–127). FcγRI has a relatively high affinity for monomeric IgG and has three immunoglobulin-like domains in the external portion of the IgG-binding chain. FcγRII and FcγRIII have a low affinity for monomeric IgG and have only two immunoglobulin-like domains in their IgG-binding chains (126, 127). Recent molecular cloning studies suggest that each class of FcγR contains more than one member (126).

Cross-linking of FcγRIII on NK cells by ligand results in an increase in $[Ca^{2+}]_i$ that is mediated by IP_3 generated from receptor-dependent hydrolysis of PIP_2 (128). Aggregation of FcγRIII on NK cells also results in activation of a nonreceptor PTK (129). Therefore, the FcγRIII-mediated hydrolysis of PIP_2 in NK cells may also be mediated by phosphorylation of PLC-γ_1 on tyrosine residues. Common features of the four receptors, mIgM, TCR, $Fc_\varepsilon RI$, and FcγRIII, all of which are functionally linked to nonreceptor tyrosine kinases, include relatively short cytoplasmic domains of the ligand-binding chains and noncovalent association of the ligand-binding chains with disulfide-linked dimers (111, 126, 127). The disulfide-linked dimer identified in the TCR is either a homodimer or a heterodimer composed of two closely related polypeptide chains, ξ and η (130, 131). The ligand-binding chain of FcγRIII in NK cells is physically associated with ξξ, ξγ, or γγ dimers (126, 127, 132), whereas only the γγ homodimer is associated with $Fc_\varepsilon RI$ (126, 133). The mIgM complex also contains a disulfide-linked heterodimer of two polypeptides encoded by the *mb1* and *b29* genes, which exhibit a limited homology to ξ, γ, and η chains (111). The ξ, γ, and η dimer-forming polypeptides possess short extracellular domains but substantial intracellular domains, and the latter are believed to play a central role in transmembrane signaling by interacting with transducing molecules (134, 135).

Despite the considerable sequence homology and similar immunoglobulin-like domain structure in the extracellular portions of the ligand-binding chains of the three classes of FcγR, the intracellular portions of the ligand-binding chains FcγRI and FcγRII are significantly different from that of FcγRIII. FcγRI and FcγRII have relatively long and highly charged cytoplasmic regions compared to FcγRIII. Furthermore, there is no evidence that FcγRI and FcγRII are associated with other subunits (127). Nevertheless, cross-linking of either FcγRI or FcγRII in monocytes elicits a rise in $[Ca^{2+}]_i$ (136–138). Liao *et al.* (139) recently observed that cross-linking of either FcγRI or FcγRII in U937 cells resulted in a rapid rise in the concentration of IP_3 as well as in a rapid and transient phosphorylation of PLC-γ_1 on tyrosine residues. Prior incubation of U937 cells with herbimycin A prevented the tyrosine phosphorylation of PLC-γ_1 as well as the hydrolysis of PIP_2 induced by the cross-linking of FcγRs. Thus, both FcγRI and FcγRII appear to be functionally coupled to a nonreceptor tyrosine kinase that phosphorylates PLC-γ_1 after receptor cross-linking, thereby causing activation of PLC-γ_1.

Prospective

Eight different isoforms of PLC have been identified in mammalian tissues and the number is certain to increase. Comparison of amino acid sequences indicates that these isoforms can be divided into three PLC types—PLC-β, γ, and δ—and that each type contains several members.

One of the important questions in signal transduction research concerns the physiological significance of the existence of multiple forms of proteins that ultimately carry out identical functions. For PLC, this question can be partially addressed by the finding that there are at least two distinct mechanisms for PLC activation: activation of PLC-β_1 and PLC-γ_1 is achieved specifically through G_q, a pertussis toxin-insensitive G protein, and through phosphorylation by protein tyrosine kinases, respectively. In many cells G protein-mediated PLC activation is pertussis toxin sensitive, indicating the involvement of a distinct G protein. As PLC-δ_1 has been shown not to be activated by G_q, members of the PLC-δ type may be effectors of such a G protein.

A single cell type can contain more than one member of the same type of PLC; for example, most leukocytes contain PLC-γ_1 and PLC-γ_2. PLC-γ_2 is also a substrate of protein tyrosine kinases. As G_q actually appears to represent a class of several proteins, such as G_{11}, G_{14}, and G_{16}, it is likely that some of these proteins activate PLC-β_2 and PLC-β_3. Thus, one can speculate about selective interactions between particular members of the PLC-β type and members of the G_q class of proteins or between particular members of the PLC-γ type and different PTKs. One can also speculate that multiple isoforms of a protein are designed to confer cells with the capability to respond differently to a variety of regulatory signals. There are numerous examples of PLC activity being affected by phorbol ester (PKC) or cAMP (PKA). Responses of PLC activity to these signaling systems vary from inhibition to activation not only between different cells but also in the same cells. Some of these diverse responses may be attributable to variation in the amino acid sequences, especially in the phosphorylation sites, between different PLC isoforms. Future research should include investigation into the significance of multiple forms of PLC in relation to the responses of PI signaling to other second messenger signaling cascades.

References

1. Carpenter, G. (1987). *Annu. Rev. Biochem.* **56,** 881–914.
2. Ullrich, A., and Schlessinger, J. (1990). *Cell* **81,** 203–212.

3. O'Dowd, B. F., Lefkowitz, R. J., and Caron, M. J. (1989). *Annu. Rev. Neurosci.* **12,** 67–83.
4. Cattaneo, M. G., and Vicentini, L. M. (1989). *Biochem. J.* **262,** 665–668.
5. Hasegawa-Sasaki, H., Lutz, F., and Sasaki, T. (1988). *J. Biol. Chem.* **263,** 12970–12976.
6. Blakeley, D. M., Corps, A. N., and Brown, K. D. (1989). *Biochem. J.* **258,** 177–185.
7. Johnson, R. M., and Garrison, J. C. (1987). *J. Biol. Chem.* **262,** 17285–17293.
8. Hepler, J. R., Jeffs, R. A., Huckle, W. R., Outlaw, H. E., Rhee, S. G., and Earp, H. S. (1990). *Biochem. J.* **270,** 337–344.
9. Huang, C. L., and Ives, H. E. (1989). *J. Biol Chem.* **264,** 4391–4397.
10. Kubo, T., Fukuda, K., Mikami, A., Maeda, A., Takahash, H., Mishina, M., Haga, T., Haga, K., Ichiyama, A., Kangawa, K., Kojima, M., Matsuo H., Hirose, T., and Numa, S. (1986). *Nature (London)* **232,** 411–416.
11. Peralta, E. G., Winslow, J. W., Peterson, G. L., Smith, D. H., Ashkenazi, A., Ramachandran, J., Schimerlik, M. I., and Capon, D. J. (1987). *Science* **236,** 600–605.
12. Bonner, T. I., Buckley, N. J., Young, A. C., and Brann, M. R. (1987). *Science* **237,** 527–532.
13. Peralta, E. G., Ashkenazi, A., Winslow, J. W., Ramachandran, J., and Capon, D. J. (1988). *Nature (London)* **334,** 434–437.
14. Liao, C. F., Themmen, A. P., Joho, R., Baberis, C., and Birnbaumer, M. (1989). *J. Biol. Chem.* **264,** 7328–7337.
15. Conklin, B. R., Brann, M. R., Buckley, N. J., Ma, A. L., Bonner, T. I., and Axelrod, J. (1988). *Proc. Natl. Acad. Sci. U.S.A.* **85,** 8698–8702.
16. Fukuda, K., Higashida, H., Kubo, T., Maeda, A., Akiba, I., Bujo, H., Mishina, M., and Numa, S. (1988). *Nature (London)* **335,** 355–358.
17. Ashkenazi, A., Winslow, J. W., Peralta, E. G., Peterson, G. L., Schimerlik, M. I., Capon, D. J., and Ramachandran, J. (1987). *Science* **238,** 672–674.
18. Bizzarri, C., Di Girolamo, M., D'Orazio, M. C., and Corda, D. (1990). *Proc. Natl. Acad. Sci. U.S.A.* **87,** 4889–4893.
19. Anderson, P. H., Gingrich, J. A., Bates, M. D., Dearry, A., Falardeau, P., Senogles, S. E., and Caron, M. G. (1990). *Trends Pharmacol. Sci.* **11,** 231–236.
20. Vallar, L., Vicentini, L. M., and Meldolesi, J. (1988). *J. Biol. Chem.* **263,** 10127–10134.
21. Bockaert, J., Journot, L., and Engalbert, A. (1988). *J. Recept. Res.* **8,** 225–243.
22. Rhee, S. G., Suh, P. G., Ryu, S. H., and Lee, S. Y. (1989). *Science* **244,** 546–550.
23. Henner, D. J., Yang, M., Chen, E., Hellmiss, R., Rodriguez, H., and Low, M. G. (1988). *Nucleic Acids Res.* **16,** 10383.
24. Kuppe, A., Evans, L. M., McMillen, D. A., and Griffith, O. H. (1989). *J. Bacteriol.* **171,** 6077–6083.
25. Stahl, M. L., Ferenz, C. R., Kelleher, K. L., Kriz, R. W., and Knopf, J. L. (1988). *Nature (London)* **332,** 369–272.
26. Suh, P. G., Ryu, S. H., Moon, K. H., Suh, H. W., and Rhee, S. G. (1988). *Proc. Natl. Acad. Sci. U.S.A.* **85,** 5419–5423.
27. Suh, P. G., Ryu, S. H., Moon, K. H., Suh, H. W., and Rhee, S. G. (1988). *Cell* **54,** 161–169.
28. Katan, M., Kriz, R. W., Totty, N., Philp, R., Meldrum, E., Aldape, R. A., Knopf, J. L., and Parker, P. J. (1988). *Cell* **54,** 171–177.
29. Bennett, C. F., Balcarek, J. M., Varrichio, A., and Crooke, S. T. (1988). *Nature (London)* **334,** 268–270.
30. Emari, Y., Homma, Y., Sarimachi, H., Kawasaki, H., Nakanish, O., Suzuki, K., and Takenawa, T. (1989). *J. Biol. Chem.* **264,** 21885–21890.
31. Ryu, S. H., Cho, K. Y., Suh, P. G., and Rhee, S. G. (1986). *Biochem. Biophys. Res. Commun.* **141,** 137–144.
32. Ryu, S. H., Cho, K. S., Lee, K. Y., Suh, P. G., and Rhee, S. G. (1987). *J. Biol. Chem.* **262,** 12511–12518.

33. Ryu, S. H., Suh, P. G., Cho, K. S., Lee, K. Y., and Rhee, S. G. (1987). *Proc. Natl. Acad. Sci. U.S.A.* **84,** 6649–6653.
34. Katan, M., and Parker, P. J. (1987). *Eur. J. Biochem.* **168,** 413–418.
35. Lips, D. L., Majerus, P. W., Gorga, F. R., Young, A. T., and Benjamin, T. L. (1989). *J. Biol. Chem.* **264,** 98759–98763.
36. Serunian, L. A., Haber, M. T., Fukui, T., Kim, J. W., Rhee, S. G., Lowenstein, J. M., and Cantley, L. C. (1989). *J. Biol. Chem.* **264,** 17809–17815.
37. Wilson, D. B., Bross, T. E., Sherman, W. R., Berger, R. A., and Majerus, P. W. (1985). *Proc. Natl. Acad. Sci. U.S.A.* **82,** 4013–4017.
38. Kim, J. W., Ryu, S. H., and Rhee, S. G. (1989). *Biochem. Biophys. Res. Commun.* **163,** 177–182.
39. Ross, T. S., Whiteley, B., Graham, R. A., and Majerus, P. W. (1991). *J. Biol. Chem.* **266,** 9086–9092.
40. Kim, U. H., Kim, J. W., and Rhee, S. G. (1989). *J. Biol. Chem.* **264,** 20167–20170.
41. Rhee, S. G. (1991). *Trends Biochem. Sci.* **10,** 168–171.
42. Martin, J. L., Pumford, N. R., LaRosa, A. C., Martin, B. M., Gonzaga, H. M. S., Beaven, M. A., and Pohl, L. R. (1991). *Biochem. Biophys. Res. Commun.* **178,** 679–685.
43. Kriz, R., Lin, L. L., Sultzman, L., Ellis, C., Heldin, C. H., Pawson, T., and Knopf, J. (1990). *In* "Proto-Oncogenes in Cell Development," pp. 112–127. Wiley, Chichester (Ciba Foundation Symposium 150).
44. Bloomquist, B. T., Shortridge, R. T., Schneuwley, S., Perdew, M., Montell, C., Steller, H., Rubin, G., and Pak, W. L. (1988). *Cell* **54,** 723–733.
45. Ohta, S., Matsui, A., Nozawa, Y., and Kagawa, Y. (1988). *FEBS Lett.* **242,** 31–35.
46. Pawson, T. (1988). *Oncogene* **3,** 491–495.
47. Bristol, A., Hall, S. M., Kriz, R. W., Stahl, M. L., Fan, Y. S., Byers, M. G., Eddy, R. L., Show, T. B., and Knopf, J. L. (1990). *Cold Spring Harbor Symp. Quant. Biol.* **53,** 915–920.
48. Baker, M. E. (1989). *Mol. Cell Endrocrinol.* **61,** 129–131.
49. Clark, J. D., Lin, L. L., Kriz, R. W., Ramesha, C. S., Sultzman, L. A., Lin, A. Y., Milona, N., and Knopf, J. L. (1991). *Cell* **65,** 1043–1051.
50. Ting, A. E. and Pagano, R. E. (1990). *J. Biol Chem.* **265,** 5337–5340.
51. Gilman, A. G. (1987). *Annu. Rev. Biochem.* **56,** 615–649.
52. Strathmann, M., and Simon, M. I. (1990). *Proc. Natl. Acad. Sci. U.S.A.* **87,** 9113–9117.
53. Amatruda, T. T., Steele, D. A., Slepak, V. Z., and Simon, M. I. (1991). *Proc. Natl. Acad. Sci. U.S.A.* **88,** 5587–5591.
54. Fain, J. N., Wallace, M. A., and Wojcikiewicz, R. J. (1988). *FASEB J.* **2,** 2569–2574.
55. Cockcroft, S., and Stutchfield, J. (1988). *Philos. Trans. R. Soc. Lond. [Biol.]* **320,** 247–265.
56. Cockcroft, S., and Gomperts, B. D. (1985). *Nature (London)* **314,** 534–536.
57. Wallace, M. A., and Fain, J. N. (1985). *J. Biol. Chem.* **260,** 9527–9530.
58. Harden, T. K., Stephens, L., Hawkins, P. T., and Downes, C. P. (1987). *J. Biol. Chem.* **262,** 9057–9061.
59. Litosch, I., Wallis, C., and Fain, J. N. (1985). *J. Biol Chem.* **260,** 5464–5471.
60. Ui, M. (1984). *Trends Pharmacol. Sci.* **5,** 277–279.
61. West, R. E., Jr., Moss, J., Vaughan, M., Liu, T., and Liu, T. Y. (1985). *J. Biol. Chem.* **260,** 14428–14430.
62. Voyno-Yasenetskaya, T. A., Tkachuk, V. A., Cheknyova, E. G., Panchenko, M. P., Grigorian, G. Y., Vavrek, R. J., Stewart, J. M., and Ryan, U. S. (1989). *FASEB J.* **3,** 44–51.
63. Perney, T. M., and Miller, R. J. (1989). *J. Biol. Chem.* **264,** 7317–7327.
64. Ashkenazi, A., Peralta, E. G., Winslow, J. W., Ramachandran, J., and Capon, D. J. (1989). *Cell* **56,** 487–493.

65. Moriarty, T. M., Sealfon, S. C., Carty, D. J., Roberts, J. L., Iyengar, R., and Landau, E. M. (1989). *J. Biol. Chem.* **264,** 13524–13530.
66. Lapetina, E. G., and Reep, B. R. (1987). *Proc. Natl. Acad. Sci. U.S.A.* **84,** 2261–2265.
67. McAtee, P., and Dawson, G. (1990). *J. Biol. Chem.* **265,** 6788–6793.
68. Moriarty, T. M., Gillo, B., Carty, D. J., Premont, R. T., Landau, E. M., and Iyengar, R. (1988). *Proc. Natl. Acad. Sci. U.S.A.* **85,** 8865–8869.
69. Boyer, J. L., Waldo, G. L., Evans, T., Northrup, J. K., Downes, C. P., and Harden, T. K. (1989). *J. Biol. Chem.* **264,** 13917–13922.
70. Moriarty, T. M., Padrell, E., Carty, D. J., Omri, G., Landau, E. M., and Iyengar, R. (1990). *Nature (London)* **343,** 79–82.
71. Martin, T. F., and Kowalchyk, J. A. (1989). *J. Biol. Chem.* **264,** 20917–20922.
72. Carter, H. R., Wallace, M. A., and Fain, J. N. (1990). *Biochim. Biophys. Acta* **1054,** 119–128.
73. Lee, K. Y., Ryu, S. H., Suh, P. G., Choi, W. C., and Rhee, S. G. (1987). *Proc. Natl. Acad. Sci. U.S.A.* **84,** 5540–5554.
74. Pang, I. H., and Sternweis, P. C. (1990). *J. Biol. Chem.* **265,** 18707–18712.
75. Smrcka, A. V., Hepler, J. R., Brown, K. O., and Sternweis, P. O. (1991). *Science* **250,** 804–807.
76. Taylor, S. J., Smith, J. A., and Exton, J. H. (1990). *J. Biol. Chem.* **265,** 17150–17156.
77. Taylor, S. J., Chae, H. Z., Rhee, S. G., and Exton, J. H. (1991). *Nature (London)* **350,** 516–518.
78. Morris, A. J., Waldo, G. L., Downes, C. P., and Harden, T. K. (1990). *J. Biol. Chem.* **265,** 13501–13507.
79. Waldo, G. L., Boyer, J. L., Morris, A. J., and Harden, T. K. (1991). *J. Biol. Chem.* **266,** 14217–14225.
80. Linden, J., and Delahunty, T. M. (1989). *Trends Pharmacol. Sci.* **10,** 114–120.
81. Delahunty, T. M., Cronin, M. J., and Linden, J. (1988). *Biochem. J.* **255,** 69–77.
82. Litosch, I. (1989). *Biochem. J.* **261,** 245–251.
83. Van Geet, C., Deckmyn, H., Kienast, J., Wittevrongel, C., and Vermylen, J. (1990). *J. Biol. Chem.* **265,** 7920–7926.
84. Wahl, M. I., Sweatt, D., and Carpenter, G. (1987). *Biochem. Biophys. Res. Commun.* **142,** 688–695.
85. Hepler, J. R., Nakahata, N., Lovenberg, T. W., DiGuiseppi, J., Herman, B., Earp, H. S., and Harden, T. K. (1987). *J. Biol. Chem.* **262,** 2951–2956.
86. Whetton, A. D., Monk, P. N., Consalvey, S. D., and Downes, C. P. (1986). *EMBO J.* **5,** 3281–3286.
87. Magnaldo, I., L'Allemanin, G., Chambard, J. C., Moenner, M., Barritault, D., and Pouyssigur, J. (1986). *J. Biol. Chem.* **261,** 16916–16922.
88. Kaibuchi, K., Tsuda, T., Kikuchi, A., Tanimoto, T., Yamashita, T., and Takai, Y. (1986). *J. Biol. Chem.* **261,** 1187–1192.
89. Farse, R. V., Kuo, J. Y., Babischkin, J. S., and Davis, J. S. (1986). *J. Biol. Chem.* **261,** 8589–8592.
90. Thakker, J. K., DiMarchi, R., MacDonald, K., and Caro, J. F. (1989). *J. Biol. Chem.* **264,** 7169–7175.
91. Thomas, A. P., Martin-Reguero, A., and Williamson, J. R. (1985). *J. Biol. Chem.* **260,** 5963–5973.
92. Besterman, J. M., Watson, S. P., and Cuatrecasas, P. (1986). *J. Biol. Chem.* **261,** 723–727.
93. Moolenaar, W. H., Bierman, A. J., Tilly, B. C., Verlaan, I., Defize, L. H. K., Honegger, A. M., Ullrich, A., and Schlessinger, J. (1988). *EMBO J.* **7,** 707–710.
94. Escobedo, J. A., Barr, P. J., and Williams, L. T. (1988). *Mol. Cell Biol.* **8,** 5126–5131.

95. Margolis, B., Bellot, F., Honegger, A. M., Ullrich, A., Schlessinger, J., and Zilberstein, A. (1990a). *Mol. Cell Biol.* **10,** 435–441.
96. Wahl, M. I., Daniel, T. O., and Carpenter, G. (1988). *Science* **241,** 968–970.
97. Wahl, M. I., Nishibe, S., Suh, P. G., Rhee, S. G., and Carpenter, G. (1989). *Proc. Natl. Acad. Sci. U.S.A.* **86,** 1568–1572.
98. Wahl, M. I., Olashaw, N. E., Nishibe, S., Rhee, S. G., Pledger, W. J., and Carpenter, G. (1989). *Mol. Cell Biol.* **9,** 2934–2943.
99. Meisenhelder, J., Suh, P. G., Rhee, S. G., and Hunter, T. (1989). *Cell* **57,** 1108–1122.
100. Margolis, B., Rhee, S. G., Felder, S., Mervic, M., Lyall, R., Levitzki, A., Ullrich, A., Zilberstein, A., and Schlessinger, J. (1989). *Cell* **57,** 1101–1107.
101. Kumjian, D. A., Wahl, M. I., Rhee, S. G., and Daniel, T. O. (1989). *Proc. Natl. Acad. Sci. U.S.A.* **86,** 8232–8326.
102. Huckle, W. R., Hepler, J. R., Rhee, S. G., Harden, T. K., and Earp, H. S. (1990). *Endocrinology* **127,** 1697–1705.
103. Kumjian, D. A., Barnstein, A., Rhee, S. G., and Daniel, T. O. (1991). *J. Biol. Chem.*, in press.
104. Morrison, D. K., Kaplan, D. R., Rhee, S. G., and Williams, L. T. (1990). *Mol. Cell Biol.* **10,** 2359–2366.
105. Nishibe, S., Wahl, M. I., Wedegaertner, P. B., Kim, J. W., Rhee, S. G., and Carpenter, G. (1990). *Proc. Natl. Acad. Sci. U.S.A.* **87,** 424–428.
106. Downing, J. R., Margolis, B. L., Zilberstein, A., Ashmun, R. A., Ullrich, A., Sherr, C. J., and Schlessinger, J. (1989). *EMBO J.* **8,** 3345–3350.
107. Nishibe, S., Wahl, M. I., Rhee, S. G., and Carpenter, G. (1989). *J. Biol. Chem.* **264,** 10335–10338.
108. Kim, J. W., Sim, S. S., Kim, U. H., Nishibe, S., Wahl, M. I., Carpenter, G., and Rhee, S. G. (1990). *J. Biol. Chem.* **265,** 3940–3943.
109. Kim, H. K., Kim, J. W., Zilberstein, A., Margolis, B., Kim, J. G., Schlessinger, J., and Rhee, S. G. (1991). *Cell* **65,** 435–441.
110. Sultzman, L., Ellis, C., Lin, L. L., Pawson, T., and Knopf, J. (1991). *Mol. Cell Biol.* **11,** 2018–2025.
111. Campbell, K. S., Hager, E. J., Friedrich, R. J., and Cambier, J. C. (1991). *Proc. Natl. Acad. Sci. U.S.A.* **88,** 3982–3986.
112. Carter, R. H., Park, D. J., Rhee, S. G., and Fearon, D. T. (1991). *Proc. Natl. Acad. Sci. U.S.A.* **88,** 2745–2749.
113. Samelson, L. E., Phillips, A. F., Luong, E. T., and Klausner, R. D. (1990). *Proc. Natl. Acad. Sci. U.S.A.* **87,** 4358–4362.
114. Veillette, A., Bookman, M. A., Horak, E. M., and Bolen, J. B. (1988). *Cell* **55,** 301–308.
115. June, C. H., Fletcher, M. C., Ledbetter, J. A., and Samelson, L. E. (1990). *J. Immunol.* **144,** 1591–1599.
116. Mustelin, T., Coggeshall, K. M., Isakov, N., and Altman, A. (1990). *Science* **247,** 1584–1587.
117. June, C. H., Fletcher, M. C., Ledbetter, J. A., Schieven, G. L., Siegel, J. N., Phillips, A. F., and Samelson, L. E. (1990). *Proc. Natl. Acad. Sci. U.S.A.* **87,** 7722–7726.
118. Park, D. J., Rho, H. W., and Rhee, S. G. (1991). *Proc. Natl. Acad. Sci. U.S.A.* **88,** 5453–5456.
119. Weiss, A., Kovetzky, G., Schatzman, R. C., and Kadlecek, T. (1991). *Proc. Natl. Acad. Sci. U.S.A.* **88,** 5484–5488.
120. Secrist, J. P., Karnitz, L., and Abraham, R. T. (1991). *J. Biol. Chem.* **266,** 12135–12139.
121. Blank, U., Ra, C., Miller, L., White, K., Metzer, H., and Kinet, J.-P. (1989). *Nature (London)* **337,** 187–189.
122. Ali, H., Cunha-Melo, J. R., Saul, W. F., and Beaven, M. A. (1990). *J. Biol. Chem.* **265,** 745–753.

123. Saito, H., Ishizaka, K., and Ishizaka, T. (1989). *J. Immunol.* **143,** 250–258.
124. Park, D. J., Min, H. K., and Rhee, S. G. (1991). *J. Biol Chem.,* in press.
125. Unkeless, J. C., Scigliano, E., and Freedman, V. H. (1988). *Annu. Rev. Immunol.* **6,** 251–281.
126. Ravetch, J. V., and Kinet, J.-P. (1991). *Annu. Rev. Immunol.* **9,** 457–492.
127. Metzer, H. (1991). *Curr. Opin. Immunol.* **3,** 40–46.
128. Cassatella, M. A., Anegon, I., Cuturi, M. C., Griskey, P., Trinchieri, G., and Perussia, B. (1989). *J. Exp. Med.* **169,** 549–567.
129. Einspahr, K. J., Abraham, R. T., Binstadt, B. A., Uehara, Y., and Liebson, P. J. (1991). *Proc. Natl. Acad. Sci. U.S.A.* **88,** 6279–6283.
130. Baniyash, M., Garcia-Morales, P., Bonifacino, J. S., Samelson, L. E., and Klausner, R. D. (1988). *J. Biol. Chem.* **263,** 9874–9878.
131. Orloff, D. G., Ra, C., Frank, S. J., Klausner, R. D., and Kinet, J.-P. (1990). *Nature (London)* **347,** 189–191.
132. Anderson, P., Caligiuri, M., Ritz, J., and Schlossman, S. F. (1989). *Nature (London)* **341,** 159–162.
133. Blank, U., Ra, C., Miller, L., White, K., Metzger, H., and Kinet, J.-P. (1989). *Nature (London)* **337,** 187–189.
134. Irving, B. A., and Weiss, A. (1991). *Cell* **64,** 891–901.
135. Remeo, C., and Seed, B. (1991). *Cell* **64,** 1037–1046.
136. Macintyre, E. A., Roberts, P. J., Abdul-Gaffar, R., O'Flynn, K., Pilkington, G. R., Farace, F., Morgan, J., and Linch, D. C. (1988). *J. Immunol.* **141,** 4333–4343.
137. Macintyre, E. A., Roberts, P. J., Jones, M., Ven der Schoot, C. E., Favaslaro, E. J., Tidman, N., and Linch, D. C. (1989). *J. Immunol.* **142,** 2377–2383.
138. Van de Winkel, J. G. J., Tax, W. J. M., Jacobs, C. W. M., Huizinga, T. W. J., and Willems, P. H. G. M. (1990). *Scand. J. Immunol.* **31,** 315–325.
139. Liao, F., Shin, H. S., and Rhee, S. G. (1991). Submitted.

CHAPTER 4

Phosphatidylcholine Metabolism in Signal Transduction

Stephen B. Bocckino and John H. Exton

Howard Hughes Medical Institute and
Department of Molecular Physiology and Biophysics
Vanderbilt University School of Medicine
Nashville, Tennessee 37232

Introduction

Although the hepatocyte is not an inflammatory cell, there is reason to believe that many of the signaling pathways found in the hepatocyte are also present in the other types of cells described in this series. In this chapter we review our work on phosphatidylcholine (PC) breakdown and hormone action in the rat liver. These studies reflect the tremendous interest in the mechanisms of signal transduction in many laboratories today. In particular, the study of G proteins and of the breakdown of inositol phospholipids provided the basis for the work described here.

Liver as an Experimental System

The rat liver has many advantages as a system for elucidating the mechanisms of signal transduction. Approximately 10 g of liver is available from a 250-g rat; the collagenase perfusion method yields 3–4 g of hepatocytes

Cellular and Molecular Mechanisms of Inflammation, Volume 3

from each liver (1). These hepatocytes are 85–95% viable and respond to a wide variety of agonists, including epinephrine, norepinephrine, vasopressin, angiotensin II, glucagon, epidermal growth factor, insulin, and ATP. Hepatocytes can be incubated in Krebs–Henseleit buffer for about 3 hr, or can be kept in primary culture in various culture media. The intact rat liver can be perfused, and the efflux or influx of metabolites (e.g., glucose, lactate, and amino acids) can be measured. Subcellular fractions are easy to prepare from the liver by a profusion of published methods. These advantages may well arouse the envy of workers using other cell types, but the liver also has limitations as an experimental system.

Radioisotopic labeling is often not very effective, given the limited duration of viability of isolated hepatocytes, necessitating *in vivo* labeling, usually by intraperitoneal injection of large amounts of isotope at high cost. Hepatocytes lose some of their responses to hormones rather quickly in primary culture, limiting the usefulness of this approach. The abundance of biological material, coupled with the difficulty of radioisotopic labeling, led us away from isotopic methods to mass measurements and to an appreciation of the role of PC breakdown in signal transduction.

Diacylglycerol Accumulation

Diacylglycerol (DAG) was first portrayed as a second messenger in the studies conducted by Nishizuka and colleagues (2, 3), who showed that protein kinase C (PKC) could be activated by 1,2-DAG. These studies coincided with the discovery that phosphatidylinositol 4,5-bisphosphate (PIP_2), a quantitatively minor lipid in the plasma membrane, was hydrolyzed in response to hormones that elevate intracellular Ca^{2+} (4). The products of this hydrolysis were inositol 1,4,5-trisphosphate (IP_3), which mobilizes Ca^{2+} from intracellular stores (5), and DAG (Fig. 1). The theory that the hydrolysis of PIP_2 gave rise to second messengers in two diverging pathways was appealing (6, 7) and has proved very popular.

In 1984, when we began to study DAG, it was believed that this lipid accumulated transiently following stimulation by agonists and was derived from PIP_2. This belief was grounded in the theory described above (6, 7) and was supported in part by radioisotopic measurements of DAG. Since DAG was thought to be generated in very small amounts, mass measurements had been attempted only infrequently. By adapting Hamilton and Comai's (8) high-performance liquid chromatography (HPLC) separation for neutral lipids to detection by refractive index, we were able to measure 1,2-DAG in hepatocyte extracts (9). In the original method (8) ab-

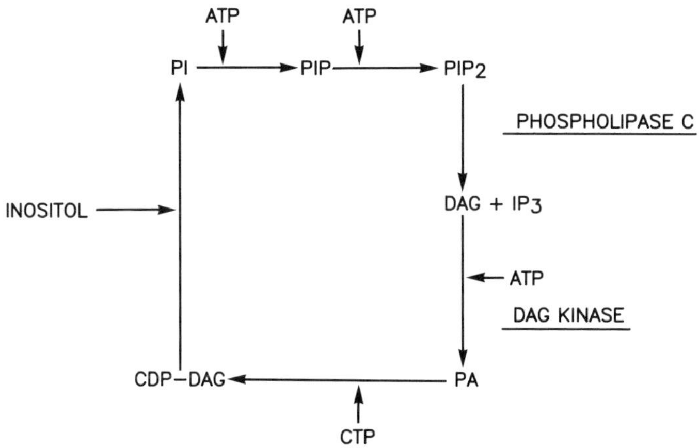

FIGURE 1

The inositol phospholipid cycle. DAG, Diacylglycerol; PA, phosphatidate; PI, phosphatidylinositol; PIP, phosphatidylinositol phosphate; PIP_2, phosphatidylinositol 4,5-bisphosphate; IP_3, inositol 1,4,5-trisphosphate.

sorbance at 206 nm was used to detect lipids, but absorbance increased greatly with unsaturation of the substituent fatty acids. Refractive index is not affected by lipid unsaturation, and changes in refractive index are linearly related to the amount of lipid. Unfortunately, refractive index detectors are sensitive to pumping irregularities and changes in ambient temperature and eluant composition, while not being particularly sensitive to DAG. These qualities did not endear the device to us. Bligh and Dyer (10) extracts from isolated hepatocytes were chromatographed over silicic acid (to remove phospholipids, which would foul the HPLC column) and injected on a μPorasil silica column (Waters, Milford, MA) (9). The column was developed isocratically with hexane:isopropanol:acetic acid (100:1: 0.01) at a flow rate of 2 ml/min. Hepatocyte 1,2-DAG eluted in 10–12.5 min in a bimodal peak following cholesterol (Fig. 2). Isomerization to 1,3-DAG, which eluted before cholesterol, was less than 5% using this method.

Vasopressin (0.1–100 n*M*) elicited DAG accumulation with an EC_{50} of 1.2 n*M*; phosphorylase was half-maximally activated by 0.09 n*M* vasopressin, reflecting increases in $[Ca^{2+}]_i$ (9) (Fig. 3). The accumulation of DAG therefore required higher concentrations of vasopressin than did Ca^{2+} mobilization. The amount of DAG in hepatocytes treated with 100 n*M* vasopressin rose from control levels of 203 ± 49 pmol/mg of wet weight to two to three times that over a period of 8 min. These quantities of DAG are equivalent to approximately 1% of the hepatocyte phospholipid.

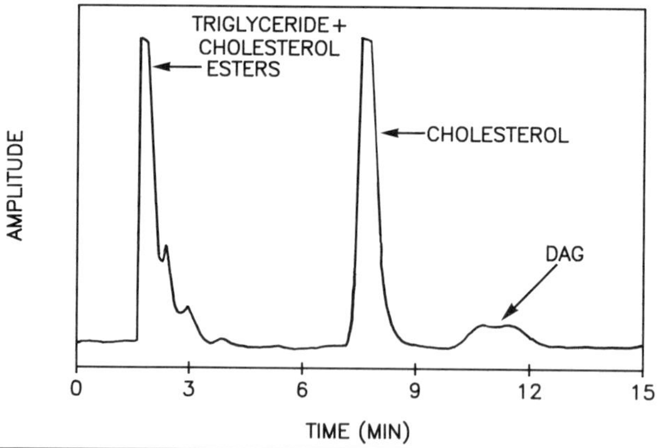

FIGURE 2

HPLC separation of diacylglycerol (DAG). Isolated hepatocytes were incubated with 10 n*M* vasopressin for 8 min. The lipids were then extracted, the phospholipids were removed by silicic acid chromatography, and the extract was chromatographed as described in the text. DAG eluted in a bimodal peak at 10–12.5 min. (Adapted from Ref. 9).

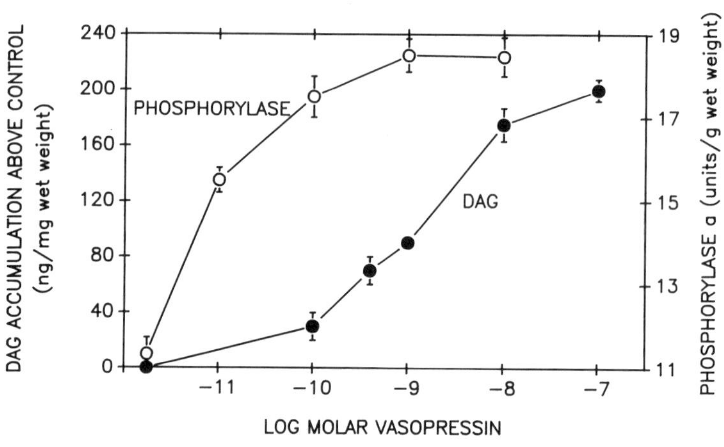

FIGURE 3

The dependence on vasopressin concentration of phosphorylase *a* activity and diacylglycerol (DAG) accumulation. Hepatocytes were incubated with the indicated concentrations of vasopressin for 8 min. Control DAG was 102 ± 6 ng/mg of wet weight. (Adapted from Ref. 9).

Epinephrine, angiotensin II, and ATP increased DAG levels by 65%, 80%, and 200%, respectively, at maximally effective hormone concentrations. DAG accumulated over about 8 min, usually after a 1- to 3-min lag, and remained elevated for at least 30 min (Fig. 4). Increases in DAG required higher concentrations of epinephrine and angiotensin II than did activation of phosphorylase (9). In contrast to the report by Farese and colleagues (11) that insulin causes a large rapid increase of DAG, we have observed an increase of only about 10% in response to this hormone (unpublished observations).

Sources of DAG

Elevations in the cellular levels of DAG can be due to increased synthesis or decreased breakdown of the lipid. Hormones may inhibit DAG lipase, DAG kinase, or DAG acyltransferase to increase DAG levels, but we have not explored these pathways. Instead, we have concentrated on the formation of DAG from phospholipids by phospholipases. One way to study the formation of DAG is by analysis of its fatty acid substituents. The fatty acid composition of hepatocyte 1,2-DAG was determined by gas chromatography of the fatty acid methyl esters (9). The DAG elicited by vasopressin (10 n*M*) at 8 min contained mainly palmitic, stearic, oleic, linoleic, and arachidonic acids. The earlier-eluting DAG peak from the HPLC col-

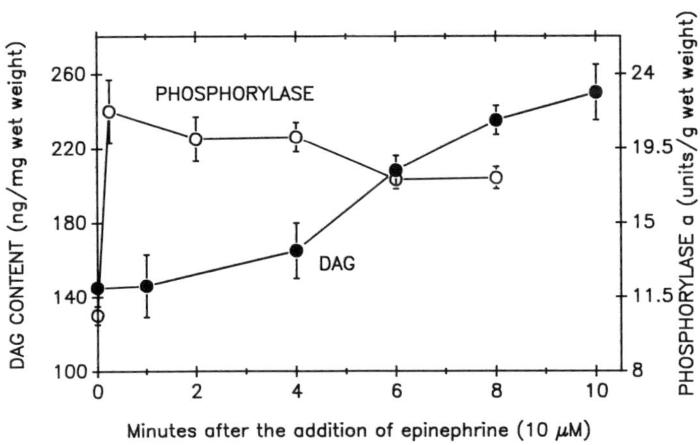

FIGURE 4

The time course of diacylglycerol (DAG) accumulation and phosphorylase activation following stimulation by epinephrine. Hepatocytes were incubated with 10 μ*M* epinephrine for the indicated times. (Adapted from Ref. 9.)

umn was enriched in stearic and arachidonic acids, while the second DAG peak was enriched in palmitic and linoleic acids. The differential elution from the HPLC column appeared to be a result of these differences in fatty acid composition. Both peaks of DAG were increased by treatment with vasopressin and ran true on repeated chromatography. The fatty acid composition of the DAG elicited by vasopressin differed from that reported for the inositol phospholipids, in which stearic and arachidonic acids usually predominate. These differences in fatty acid composition led us to believe that the DAG accumulating in response to hormones was not derived solely form the inositol phospholipids (9).

Subsequent measurements of the fatty acid composition of the inositol lipids performed in this laboratory showed that, in hepatocytes, these lipids do contain some palmitic and linoleic acids, but not enough to account for the DAG formed (12). Triglycerides, too, have a very different fatty acid composition from DAG (13). The amount of DAG formed, 130–400 pmol/mg of wet weight, also indicated that PIP_2 was not the major source, as it is present at only 19 pmol/mg of wet weight (12). Phosphorylation of PI and PIP could replenish the PIP_2 (cf. Fig. 1), but PI levels do not decline until 15 min after the addition of vasopressin (12). We interpreted these data as indicative that another lipid, perhaps PC, was the precursor of DAG. PC is present at concentrations of approximately 18 nmol/mg of wet weight of liver (14), and breakdown of only a small fraction could account for the DAG formed.

The molecular species of a particular lipid (i.e., the various molecules containing certain fatty acid substituents) convey more information than the fatty acid composition of the unfractionated lipid. The presence or absence of certain molecular species may constitute a "signature" for a particular lipid and indicate a metabolic relationship. HPLC analysis of the molecular species of DAG from hepatocytes revealed 12 major peaks (15) (Fig. 5). Vasopressin produced increases in all of these peaks, but some were increase more than others, particularly the species of DAG containing $C_{16:0}/C_{16:1}/C_{18:2}/C_{22:6}$; $C_{16:0}/C_{20:4}$; $C_{16:0}/C_{18:2}$; $C_{18:0}/C_{20:4}$; and $C_{16:0}/C_{18:1}$, $C_{18:0}/C_{18:2}$. A comparison of the molecular species observed in response to vasopressin with those of PC and PI shows that neither phospholipid gives an exact match to DAG, but that PC is the closer of the two (15) (Table I). Phosphatidylserine contains large amounts (22%) of $C_{18:0}/C_{22:6}$, which is not present in DAG; phosphatidylethanolamine is a better match than PI, but not as close as PC. We have not determined the molecular species of PIP_2, but from its fatty acid composition, it would be deficient in $C_{18:2}$-containing species compared to DAG elicited by vasopressin. The molecular species experiments, like the earlier fatty acid analyses, implicate PC as a source for this DAG (15).

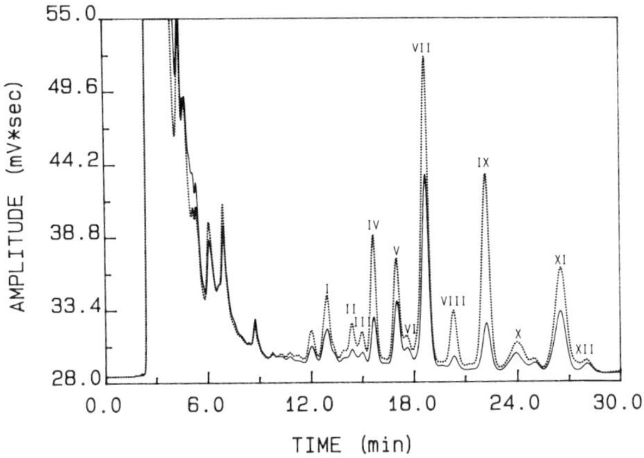

FIGURE 5

High-performance liquid chromatography (HPLC) of diacylglycerol (DAG) molecular species. Hepatocytes were incubated for 10 min with saline (solid line) or 100 n*M* vasopressin (dotted line), and the molecular species of DAG were separated by HPLC. Peaks contained (percentage of total fatty acids in a given peak is shown in parentheses): I, $C_{16:0}$ (28), $C_{16:1}$ (11), $C_{18:2}$ (32), $C_{22:6}$ (18); II, $C_{16:0}$ (37), $C_{20:4}$ (32), $C_{18:1}$ (8), $C_{18:3}$ (6); III, $C_{16:0}$ (35), $C_{18:1}$, $C_{16:0}$ (37), $C_{20:4}$ (32), $C_{18:1}$ (8), $C_{18:3}$ (6); III, $C_{16:0}$ (35), $C_{18:1}$ (10), $C_{20:4}$ (12), $C_{22:5}$ (30); IV, $C_{16:0}$ (44), $C_{20:4}$ (44); V, $C_{16:0}$ (39), $C_{18:0}$ (7), $C_{18:1}$ (7), $C_{18:2}$ (34); VI, $C_{16:0}$ (11), $C_{16:1}$ (7), $C_{18:0}$ (8), $C_{18:1}$ (37), $C_{18:2}$ (29); VII, $C_{16:0}$ (46), II, $C_{18:2}$ (43); VIII, $C_{16:0}$ (10), $C_{18:0}$ (40), $C_{18:2}$ (6), $C_{20:4}$ (36); IX, $C_{18:0}$ (46), $C_{20:4}$ (46); X, $C_{16:0}$ (29), $C_{18:0}$ (16), $C_{18:1}$ (29), $C_{18:2}$ (13), $C_{20:4}$ (7); XI, $C_{16:0}$ (31), $C_{18:0}$ (17), $C_{18:1}$ (35), $C_{18:2}$ (11); XII, $C_{16:0}$ (52), $C_{18:0}$ (17), $C_{18:1}$ (9), $C_{20:3}$ (7). (From Ref. 15.)

Effects of Phorbol Ester and Calcium Ionophore

The calcium ionophore A23187 and the phorbol ester 4β-phorbol 12β-myristate 13α-acetate (PMA) also elicited increases in DAG (9). These compounds have been used to study the effects of elevated cellular Ca^{2+} and activation of PKC, respectively. The DAG accumulation observed with A23187 suggests that a phospholipase may be activated by the rise in cytosolic Ca^{2+} elicited by hormones; however, increases in cytosolic Ca^{2+} are seen at lower concentrations of hormone than is DAG accumulation (Fig. 3). In addition depletion of cellular Ca^{2+} by incubation with the chelator EGTA inhibited only about 50% of the increase in DAG seen with vasopressin (9). These findings suggested to us that additional mechanisms mediate the increase in DAG. PMA at 1 μ*M* produced a doubling of

TABLE I

Molecular Species of DAG in Control and Vasopressin-Stimulated Hepatocytes and in Hepatocyte PC and PI[a]

	Area (arbitrary units)			% of total area		
Peak	Control DAG	VASO DAG	ΔDAG	ΔDAG	PC	PI
I	60	185	125	7.6	8.2	7.0
II	12	34	22	1.3		
III	29	75	46	2.8	5.1	3.6
IV	49	231	182	11.1	21.5	10.8
V	26	69	43	2.6		
VI	39	96	57	3.5	2.6	
VII	219	598	379	23.0	19.3	7.3
VIII	15	64	49	3.0		
IX	87	510	423	25.8	22.4	57.6
X	16	43	27	1.6		
XI	146	408	262	16.0	16.9	9.4
XII	15	40	25	1.5		
Total	713	2353	1640	99.8	96.0	95.7

[a]The DAG species correspond to those shown in Fig. 5. DAG, Diacylglycerol; PC, phosphatidylcholine; PI, phosphatidylinositol; VASO, vasopressin.

DAG levels at 8 min, indicating that PKC may activate phospholipases. In order for PKC to mediate the effects of hormones on DAG levels, the kinase itself must first be activated by DAG, raising a chicken-or-egg situation. The activating DAG may be derived from breakdown of PIP_2 in amounts too small for detection by mass measurement or by the hydrolysis of PC or other lipids stimulated by means other than PKC. While incubation with A23187 increased DAG in both HPLC peaks, PMA caused the accumulation of DAG predominantly in the later-eluting peak, enriched in palmitic and linoleic acids (9). The molecular species of DAG containing these fatty acids were also shown to accumulate, with less accumulation of $C_{18:0}/C_{20:4}$ than with other agonists. These data support the hypothesis that PMA selectively effects the hydrolysis of PC. In 1981 Mufson *et al.* (16) demonstrated that phorbol esters stimulate the hydrolysis of PC, and Grove and Schimmel (17) observed that treatment of cultured myoblasts with PMA elevated DAG levels and that the fatty acid composition of this DAG resembled that of PC. Interestingly, the phorbol esters inhibit the hydrolysis of inositol lipids in liver (18, 19), and so can serve as a tool to dissect the various pathways of hormonal breakdown of phospholipids.

In 1986 two groups published studies of phorbol esters and PC breakdown. Daniel *et al.* (20) explored PC breakdown by labeling Madin–Darby canine kidney cells with 1-*O*-[^{3}H]-alkyl-2-lysoglycero-3-phosphocholine, which is acylated by the cell to form a tritiated 1-alkyl-2-acylglycero-3-phosphocholine. They showed that treatment with PMA caused the increased synthesis of tritiated 1-alkyl-2-acylglycerol, an analog of DAG. Besterman and colleagues (21) demonstrated that, in HL-60 promyelocytes labeled with [^{14}C]oleate, phorbol dibutyrate, another phorbol ester, caused formation of [^{14}C]DAG. In 3T3-L1 preadipocytes labeled with [^{3}H]choline, phorbol dibutyrate increased the levels of [^{3}H]phosphocholine both intra- and extracellularly (21). Down-regulation of PKC by prolonged treatment with phorbol dibutyrate inhibited subsequent phosphocholine release due to phorbol ester. Platelet-derived growth factor and serum also stimulated the release of labeled phosphocholine; however, these effects were only partially blocked by down-regulation of PKC (21). These studies implicated PKC as a regulator of PC breakdown in a variety of cell types, but did not rule out other modes of regulation.

The finding that phorbol esters inhibit the breakdown of inositol phospholipids while stimulating PC breakdown has important implications (Fig. 6). DAG formed in response to agonists would stimulate PKC and terminate the hydrolysis of PIP_2 and Ca^{2+} mobilization due to IP_3. At the same time, PC hydrolysis and DAG formation would be stimulated in a positive-feedback mechanism. The two pathways would diverge temporally, the Ca^{2+} signal being short-lived and the DAG signal being sustained. This predicted pattern is observed experimentally in the hepatocyte. The long-lived DAG signal may be important in the regulation of gene expression and other events with slow time courses.

It is evident that mass measurements of DAG led to new theories about hormone action. PC, not PIP_2, appears to be the quantitatively major source of DAG, and DAG elevation is not transient. Control of DAG levels by intracellular Ca^{2+} and by PKC may mediate the actions of hormones. Dur-

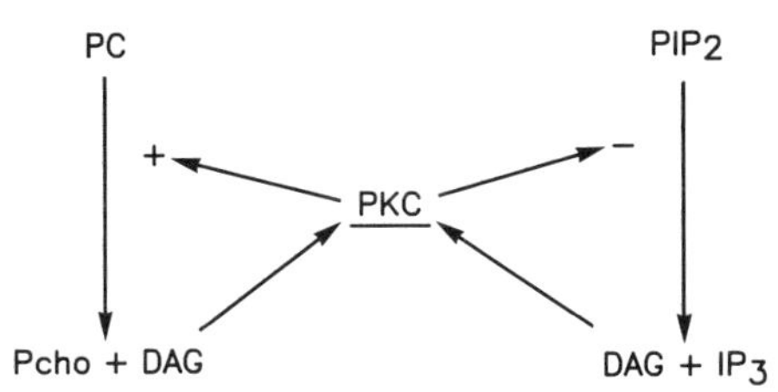

FIGURE 6

The effect of diacylglycerol (DAG) and protein kinase C (PKC) on the breakdown of phosphatidylcholine (PC) and phosphatidylinositol 4,5-bisphosphate (PIP_2). Pcho, Phosphocholine; IP_3, inositol 1,4,5-trisphosphate.

ing the HPLC studies of DAG, a more elegant and sensitive assay was developed by Preiss *et al.* (22), using DAG kinase. We were gratified that the two methods agreed within 5%, and we now use the DAG kinase assay or thin-layer chromatographic assays routinely. The HPLC method that served us so well is now relegated to preparative work.

Plasma Membrane Studies

One of the great benefits of working with liver is the easy availability of large amounts of purified plasma membranes. Irving and Exton (23) pursued the breakdown of PC in the liver plasma membrane, using a radioisotopic approach. They injected rats intraperitoneally with tritiated choline, and 18 hr later isolated liver plasma membranes from the injected animals. When they incubated the membranes with Mg^{2+}, they found that labeled material (choline plus phosphocholine) was released from the membranes. GTP and its analogs GTPγS, GMPPCP, and GMPPNP stimulated the release of labeled material, but GDPβS did not. This pattern of stimulation is seen with enzymes activated by G proteins. In addition, ATP and its analogs ATPγS and AMPPCP stimulated the release of choline plus phosphocholine. These adenine nucleotides were synergistic with submaximal concentrations of GTPγS in the release of choline and phosphocholine (Fig. 7). Vasopressin also produced a small stimulation. These findings were consistent with the hypothesis that the purinergic agonists and, to a lesser degree, vasopressin, activate a PC phospholipase C via a G protein. Since phosphocholine could not be formed from choline in these incubations, which lacked ATP, its release was indicative of phospholipase C activity. We were also able to measure the formation of the lipid product of this enzyme, DAG, under these conditions (23).

Bacterial toxins have been useful probes for G protein function. Cholera toxin catalyzes the ADP ribosylation of the α subunit of G_s, the guanine nucleotide-binding protein that activates adenylate cyclase. This modification causes great increases in cellular cAMP levels due to the persistent activation of adenylate cyclase. The islet-activating protein of pertussis toxin ADP-ribosylates the α subunit of several G proteins, including that which inhibits adenylate cyclase, G_i. This modification causes increases in cAMP, due to removal of inhibition of adenylate cyclase by G_i. Neither of these toxins, when injected into the rat, had an effect on choline plus phosphocholine release in isolated plasma membranes. These experiments appeared to preclude a role for G_s or G_i in the activation of choline plus phosphocholine release by GTPγS (23).

The activation by the adenine nucleotides required Ca^{2+}, and most of the experiments were conducted at 400 n*M* free Ca^{2+}. The possibility that the

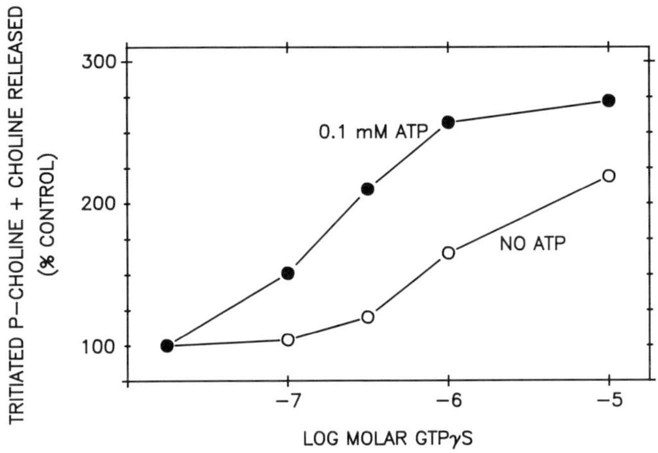

FIGURE 7

The effect of GTPγS and ATP on the release of tritiated choline and phosphocholine (P-CHOLINE) from labeled rat liver plasma membranes. Rats were injected intraperitoneally with tritiated choline, and plasma membranes were isolated 18 hr later. Membranes were incubated at 30°C for 5 min with 10 m*M* Mg^{2+} and the indicated concentrations of GTPγS and ATP. (From Ref. 23.)

nucleotides were acting as purinergic agonists was examined using a series of agonists and antagonists. The order of potency for PC breakdown was ATPγS > ATP, ADP, AMPPNP, AMPPCP > adenosine, AMP, and αβmATP, with the order of efficacy ATPγS > ATP > ADP > AMPPNP, AMPPCP > AMP > αβmATP > adenosine. The P_2-purinergic antagonist αβmATP caused some release of labeled choline and phosphocholine, but also inhibited release due to ATP, thus acting as a partial agonist in this system. The P_2-purinergic antagonist 2,2′-pyridylisatogen (0.2 m*M*) inhibited release by 42% in the presence of 0.1 m*M* ATP and 0.3 μ*M* GTPγS. The P_1-purinergic antagonists phentolamine and quinidine, both at 0.2 m*M*, inhibited release by only 12%. These data support a P_2-purinergic mechanism for the breakdown of PC in the liver plasma membrane (23).

The tumor promoter PMA also elicited release of labeled choline and phosphocholine from liver plasma membranes. PMA has been shown to activate PKC and increased the release of label from the plasma membranes in the presence of ATP and GTPγS. The effect of PMA could be seen without added Ca^{2+}, but not at higher Ca^{2+}, when the P_2-purinergic effects predominated (23). These data are suggestive of activation of PC breakdown in the plasma membrane by PKC that is separate from the receptor-mediated purinergic effect.

Phosphatidate Accumulation

In many cell types phosphatidate (PA) accumulates in response to agonists. Originally, it was thought that this PA was formed by the action of DAG kinase on DAG formed by phospholipase C acting on inositol phospholipids. This PA was then channeled back into inositol lipids, forming a cycle (Fig. 1). An alternative view was expressed by Hokin-Neaverson (24) and by Cockcroft (25), who presented evidence for a phospholipase D acting on PI. There had been very few measurements of cellular PA in stimulated cells, and most workers relied on estimates of turnover, using ^{32}P labeling. We developed a thin-layer chromatography method, using two different solvent systems in the same dimension that resolved PA from the other phospholipids (26). Coomassie Blue, which stains lipids in addition to proteins (27), was used to visualize the PA in the range of 0.1–2 μg. The plates were then scanned, using a densitometer, and the results were compared with a standard curve of PA run on every plate. This method provided the selectivity and sensitivity required to measure PA in lipid extracts from hepatocytes.

PA levels rose quickly in hepatocytes treated with vasopressin and peaked before DAG did (26) (Fig. 8). This finding was at odds with the theory that DAG was the precursor of PA via DAG kinase. The fatty acid composition of both PA and DAG changed upon hormonal stimulation, but the changes in PA were evident first. The DAG kinase inhibitors ethylene glycol dioctanoate (28) and R59 022 (29) did not affect PA or DAG levels in the presence or absence of vasopressin. Again, the data disagreed with the concept that PA was formed by DAG kinase. It has been suggested recently that the DAG in neutrophils and HL-60 granulocytes is derived from PA by the action of PA phosphohydrolase (30) (Fig. 9). Our data are consistent with this model, but we also have evidence of a PC phospholipase C pathway acting in hepatocytes (see "Plasma Membrane Studies" under "Phosphatidate Accumulation"), which may be a source of DAG. Vasopressin elicited similar amounts of PA and DAG, a total equivalent to 1–2% of the hepatocyte phospholipid. This PA and DAG remained associated with the hepatocyte (unpublished observations) and was not secreted, as observed by Murayama and Ui (31) in the thrombin-stimulated rabbit platelet.

The other Ca^{2+}-mobilizing agonists, angiotensin II, epinephrine, ATP, and epidermal growth factor, also raised PA levels within minutes (26). In

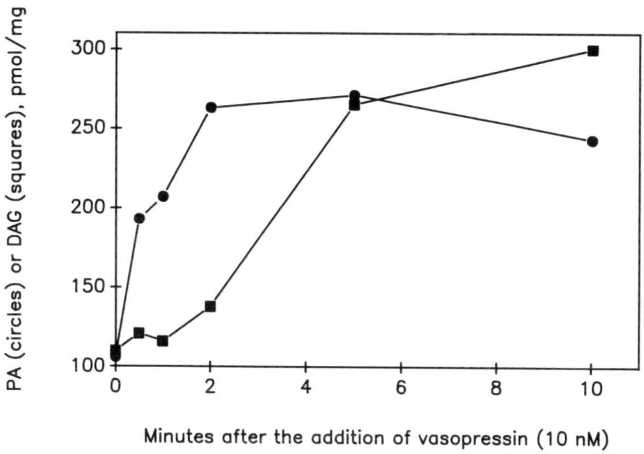

FIGURE 8

Time course of phosphatidate (PA) and diacylglycerol (DAG) accumulation in hepatocytes stimulated with vasopressin. Hepatocytes were incubated with 10 n*M* vasopressin for the indicated times. (Redrawn from Ref. 26.)

hepatocytes all of the known Ca^{2+}-mobilizing agonists increased the concentrations of PA and DAG. Thus far we have found no agonist that increases PA and DAG levels that does not also mobilize Ca^{2+}, with the exception of exogenously added phospholipases. We are uncertain whether this is a peculiarity of liver or whether it reflects an important coupling of the pathways. In some cultured cell lines growth factors can increase DAG levels without an increase in cytosolic Ca^{2+} (32), but this may be a result of changes in culture. Alternatively, certain agonists may increase

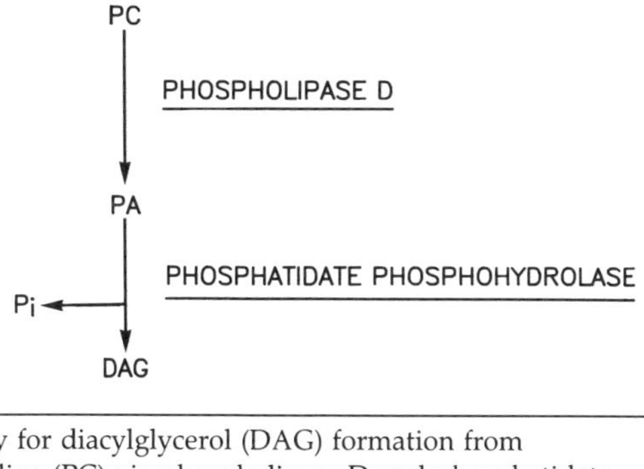

FIGURE 9

Possible pathway for diacylglycerol (DAG) formation from phosphatidylcholine (PC) via phospholipase D and phosphatidate (PA) phosphohydrolase. P_i, Inorganic phosphate.

cellular levels of PA or DAG, but not Ca^{2+}, as an intrinsic feature of their signaling pathway.

Plasma Membrane Studies

To explore the mechanism of PA formation, we took advantage of the liver plasma membrane system, which had been used previously to examine the breakdown of polyphosphoinositides and PC in our laboratory (33). When a washed plasma membrane preparation was incubated with Mg^{2+} at 37°C, PA was formed for about 10 min after a 1- to 2-min lag (26) (Fig. 10). When GTPγS, a poorly hydrolyzable analog of GTP, was included in the incubation, more PA was formed. The reaction was half-maximally stimulated by 1.5 μ*M* GTPγS, and so was similar to reactions stimulated by G proteins. The activation by GTPγS was blocked by GDPβS, a GDP analog. These findings were consistent with a process regulated by a G protein.

Aluminum fluoride, which activates G proteins, is another tool commonly used in G protein research. This salt caused a profound inhibition of PA formation in the plasma membrane preparation, even in the presence of excess Mg^{2+} (magnesium fluoride is poorly soluble). Aluminum fluoride seems to have a direct inhibitory effect on the formation of PA, although we have not ruled out the presence of an inhibitory G protein. We originally reported that aluminum fluoride was without effect on PA

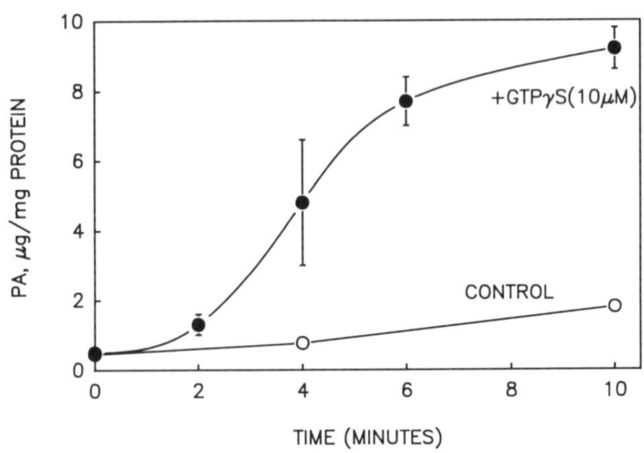

FIGURE 10

The effect of GTPγS on phosphatidate (PA) formation by rat liver plasma membranes. Plasma membranes were incubated for the indicated times with 10 m*M* Mg^{2+} and water or 10 μ*M* GTPγS. (From Ref. 26.)

levels in intact hepatocytes, and we proposed that it might be useful in dissecting out the role of PA in hormonal responses (26). In later experiments with higher concentrations of fluoride and longer time courses (unpublished observations), we have observed accumulation of PA in intact hepatocytes. This effect of fluoride in intact cells was not blocked by desferoxamine, a high-affinity chelator of aluminum, which may indicate that fluoride is not acting through a G protein in intact cells. Thus fluoride has not proved as useful as we had hoped.

Cholera toxin, which modifies the α subunit of G_s, and pertussis toxin, which modifies G_i, were without effect on the amount of PA elicited by vasopressin in intact hepatocytes (26). These holotoxins require activation by the cell in order to become active, but the α subunits of the toxins do not require activation and can be used in cell-free preparations. The α subunits of the toxins had no effect on PA levels in the plasma membrane preparations, in the presence or absence of GTPγs. These incubations were performed with NAD, which is necessary for the ADP ribosylation reactions catalyzed by the toxins. Again, it appeared that neither G_s nor G_i is involved in PA production.

The accumulation of PA in plasma membranes did not require the addition of ATP, and incubation with [^{32}P]ATP did not lead to incorporation of the label into PA. Formation of PA by the action of DAG kinase was thus excluded. An alternative pathway for PA production was by phospholipase D. A phospholipase D activity producing PA from PI had been described previously by Hokin-Neaverson (24) and by Cockcroft (25). Taki and Kanfer (34) described and partially purified a phospholipase D in rat brain acting on PC. Phospholipase D had been studied primarily in plants and, prior to Taki and Kanfer's work, many biochemists had believed that animals did not possess this enzyme. It has been argued that, even in plants, the phospholipase D was not active *in vivo* (35). The cellular function of phospholipase D was unknown. The PI phospholipase D activity was stimulated by agonists, but the PC-hydrolyzing activity had not been investigated in this regard. When liver plasma membranes were incubated with the chelator EGTA, which blocked the breakdown of the inositol lipids (33), the accumulation of PA was reduced by about one-third (26). This inhibition was reversed by the addition of sufficient Ca^{2+} to achieve a calculated free Ca^{2+} of 72 n*M*. We incubated plasma membranes with EGTA and Mg^{2+}, with or without GTPγS, for 10 min and separated the lipids by two-dimensional thin-layer chromatography. The phospholipids were then measured by phosphorus analysis; PC was the only phospholipid to break down under these conditions, and the amount of breakdown in incubations containing GTPγS was more than enough to account for the PA produced in the experiment (Table II). This was a clear demonstration that the membranes contained a phospholipase D activity acting on PC and stimulated by GTPγS (26).

To confirm this finding, we measured the release of choline and phosphocholine mass using the choline kinase assay (26). When plasma membranes were incubated with GTPγS and Mg^{2+}, both choline and phosphocholine were released (Fig. 11A), in amounts similar to the PC breakdown measured by phosphorus analysis above (Table II). The release of choline and phosphocholine paralleled the formation of PA and DAG in the same experiment (Fig. 11B). This experiment demonstrated the presence of both phospholipase D and C activities in the plasma membrane. Since ATP was not included in the incubation, the presence of PA and choline is indicative of a phospholipase D. Similarly, the presence of both DAG and phosphocholine is indicative of a phospholipase C, confirming the work by Irving and Exton (23) described above. The absolute amount of choline and phosphocholine formed (and of PC breakdown) was greater than DAG plus PA formation (Fig. 11 and Table II); this may result from breakdown of DAG and PA during the incubation or from activation of other phospholipases (e.g., A_2) by GTPγS.

We attempted to show a hormonal activation of this phospholipase D (26). In previous work with the membrane system, it had been shown that Ca^{2+}-mobilizing hormones could stimulate the hydrolysis of PIP_2 in the presence of Ca^{2+} and a subsaturating amount of GTPγS (33). Under these conditions only ATP and ADP were effective in stimulating phospholipase D activity. Vasopressin, angiotensin II, and epinephrine were without significant effect. The effect of ATP was not a result of phosphorylation, as ADP was equally effective. It appears that the adenine nucleotides act

TABLE II

Effects of GTPγS on Phospholipid Levels in Hepatic Plasma Membranes[a]

GTPγS	SM	PC	PS ± PI	PA	PE
–	54.4 ± 5.8	146.3 ± 19.3	73.9 ± 6.8	3.8 ± 1.1	69.9 ± 8.9
+	56.3 ± 7.4	130.2 ± 17.2[a]	77.2 ± 5.3	11.6 ± 0.6[b]	71.4 ± 7.7

[a]Plasma membranes were incubated with or without 20 μ*M* GTPγS in the absence of added Ca^{2+} for 10 min. The phospholipids were separated by two-dimensional thin-layer chromatography and analyzed for PO_4. Values are expressed as nanomoles per milligram of protein and are the means ± SE of four separate experiments conducted in triplicate. SM, Sphingomyelin; PC, phosphatidylcholine; PS, phosphatidylserine; PI, phosphatidylinositol; PA, phosphatidate; PE, phosphatidylethanolamine. (From Ref. 26.)
[b]Different from control ($p < 0.01$, paired t test).

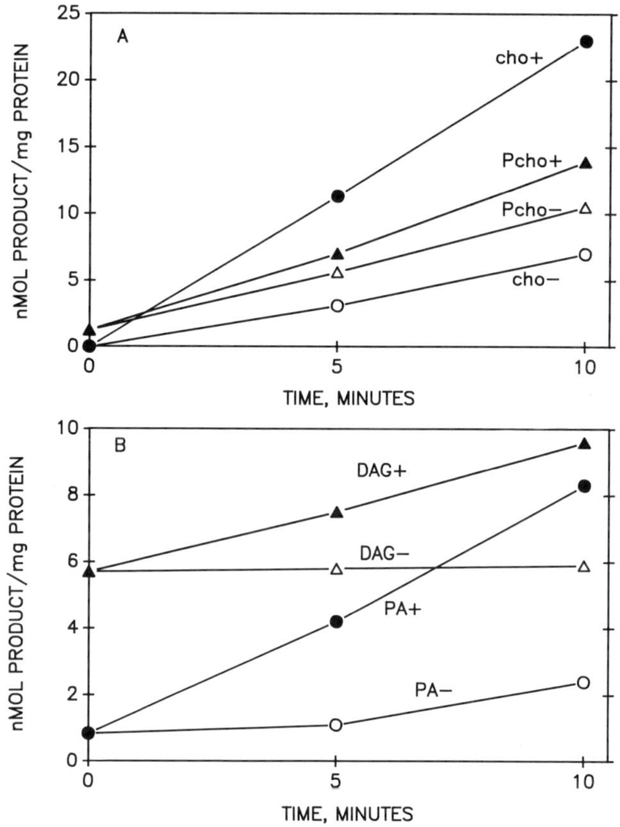

FIGURE 11

The effect of GTPγS on the production of choline (cho), phosphocholine (Pcho), phosphatidate (PA), and diacylglycerol (DAG) by plasma membranes. (A) Choline and phosphocholine were measured by the choline kinase assay after incubation of plasma membranes for the indicated times with (+) or without (−) 20 μ*M* GTPγS. (B) DAG and PA were measured by thin-layer chromatography. (From Ref. 26.)

through a P_2-purinergic receptor, which has been described in the rat liver (see "Plasma Membrane Studies" under "Diacylglycerol Accumulation"). As yet we have no insight into the lack of efficacy of the other Ca^{2+}-mobilizing hormones, but it may be that, in liver, only the purinergic receptor is coupled to the phospholipase D directly via a G protein. The other agonists may activate the phospholipase by other mechanisms or may elevate PA through other pathways.

Phosphatidylethanol Formation

Another means of estimating phospholipase D activity is by the formation of phosphatidylethanol. It has long been known that the plant phospholipases D can catalyze a transphosphatidylation reaction in addition to the usual hydrolytic reaction (36) (Fig. 12). In transphosphatidylation an alcohol reacts with PC to form a phosphatidylalcohol. Short-chain alcohols (e.g., ethanol) have been used most frequently, but the transphosphatidylation reaction has been used in the synthesis of other phosphatidyl compounds. Phospholipase D is the only enzyme reported to form phosphatidylethanol, and the formation of the lipid is taken as a measure of phospholipase D activity (30). Another advantage of measuring phosphatidylethanol is that the lipid is virtually undetectable in the absence of ethanol, providing a low background. When hepatocytes were treated with ethanol and vasopressin, angiotensin II, or epinephrine, phosphatidylethanol was formed (37) (Fig. 13). This was the first demonstration of a hormonal stimulation of phosphatidylethanol formation; previous studies had shown an effect of phorbol esters (38). Phosphatidylethanol synthesis in plasma membranes could be stimulated with GTPγS, and transphosphatidylation (i.e., phosphatidylethanol formation) was competitive with hydrolysis (i.e., PA formation) (37).

The experiments with phosphatidylethanol lent support to the hypothesis that phospholipase D is activated by hormones in hepatocytes. We have since found that phosphatidylethanol is more resistant than is PA to

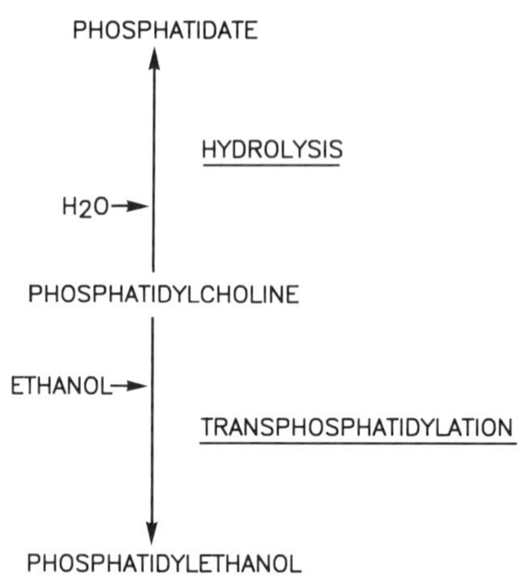

FIGURE 12

Transphosphatidylation and hydrolysis catalyzed by phospholipase D.

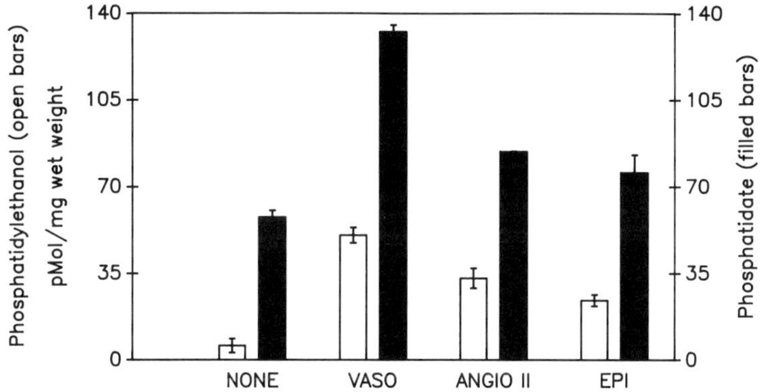

FIGURE 13

Effect of Ca^{2+}-mobilizing hormones on phosphatidylethanol and phosphatidate accumulation in rat hepatocytes. Hepatocytes were incubated for 20 min with (for phosphatidylethanol) or without (for phosphatidate) 70 m*M* ethanol followed by 10 min with the indicated hormone [100 n*M* vasopressin (VASO), 100 n*M* angiotensin II (ANGIO II), or 10 μ*M* epinephrine (EPI)]. Phosphatidylethanol and phosphatidate were quantitated by thin-layer chromatography and densitometry. (Data from Ref. 37.)

hydrolysis by detergent-activated membrane PA phosphohydrolase (unpublished observations). The assumption that phosphatidylethanol is not a good substrate for PA phosphohydrolase has spawned experiments in which the suppression of hormone-elicited DAG by high concentrations of ethanol is taken as evidence of DAG formation from PA via this enzyme. The pathway would then involve PA formation from PC by phospholipase D, followed by DAG formation from PA by PA phosphohydrolase (Fig. 9). Evidence is accumulating that this pathway may be important in some cell types, but caution must be exercised regarding the effects of high concentrations (typically 200–400 m*M*) of ethanol. Mueller and colleagues (39) have shown that white blood cells from male alcoholics can synthesize more phosphatidylethanol than can those from normal controls. This may indicate that induction of phospholipase D is a marker for excessive alcohol consumption or predisposition to alcoholism, but hormonal effects on phospholipase D should be kept in mind in this context.

Properties of the Plasma Membrane Phospholipase D

The phospholipase D of rat liver plasma membranes appears to be an intrinsic membrane protein, as it is not removed by treatment with high concentrations of salt or by chelators. Detergents of widely varying structures are uniformly inhibitory to the membrane activity, often at concentrations below the critical micellar concentration. This inhibition is not reversed by removal of the detergents by dialysis or gel filtration. The phospholipase D activity requires Mg^{2+}, other divalent cations being ineffective. This may be partially a result of a requirement for the Mg^{2+} salt of GTPγS for activation. Ca^{2+} activates by about 33% in the range of 74 n*M* to 50 μ*M*, but is inhibitory above this range. The addition of purified calmodulin, or the calmodulin-dependent protein kinase II plus calmodulin and ATP, did not activate the phospholipase D in the presence of Ca^{2+}. It appears that the Ca^{2+} requirement may be intrinsic to the enzyme or may be due to the presence of multiple forms of phospholipase D. We have not observed large activations of membrane phospholipase D by Ca^{2+} that could explain the large PA accumulation in hepatocytes treated with the Ca^{2+} ionophore A23187 (26).

Many compounds are inhibitory to the phospholipase D activity, including fluoride, diethyl ether, oleate, chlorpromazine, and propranolol (unpublished observations), all of which have been useful in the study of phospholipase D from other tissues and species. The pH optimum for the phospholipase is approximately 7.5, with very little activity detected below pH 7.0. The brain enzyme, studied by Chalifour and Kanfer (40), was optimally active at pH 6.5 in the presence of 50 m*M* fluoride and 10 m*M* EDTA. The enzyme from liver plasma membranes is totally inactive under these conditions and may be another isoenzyme. The rat brain enzyme is inactive using conditions that are optimal for the liver enzyme, and we have been unable to show stimulation of the brain enzyme by GTPγS (unpublished observations).

In Vivo Measurements of DAG and PA in the Regenerating Liver

The concentrations of hormones that increase PA and DAG in hepatocytes are higher than those elevating $[Ca^{2+}]_i$ (9, 26, 41). For example, vasopressin half-maximally activated phosphorylase at 0.09 n*M*, but PA and DAG accumulation was half-maximal at about 1.2 n*M*. Similar discrepancies are observed for epinephrine and angiotensin II. The circulating levels of these hormones are far below the concentrations needed to elicit increases in PA and DAG; the blood vasopressin level is approximately 2.5–40 p*M* (42). Glucagon greatly potentiates all of the Ca^{2+}-mobilizing hormones (43), but the accumulation of DAG and PA requires high concentrations of hormone even in the presence of glucagon (9, 26). It may be argued that noradrenergic neurons impinging on the liver provide sufficient hormone to elicit PA and DAG, but we have not yet examined this. It should be pointed out that virtually all of the work on agonist effects on DAG and PA had been done with isolated or cultured cells, and the possibility remained that increases in PA and DAG do not occur *in vivo.*

To explore the relevance of DAG and PA *in vivo,* we chose to examine a fascinating biological phenomenon: the regenerating liver. When two-thirds of a rat's liver is removed, the remaining lobes hypertrophy to restore the original mass of the liver in about 2 weeks (44). The liver, which is usually quiescent, undergoes a vigorous proliferation and exhibits large increases in DNA synthesis. What is equally interesting is that there is a return to quiescence just at the point when the original mass is restored. The partially hepatectomized rat has been studied by numerous workers, but despite their efforts, the mechanisms controlling regeneration are not yet known. Both PA (45–47) and DAG (48) are mitogens for certain cultured cells; that is, they increase the incorporation of tritiated thymidine into DNA, actually a measure of DNA synthesis and not mitogenicity per se. We wanted to determine whether these lipids played any part in the regeneration of liver. In preliminary experiments we found that variability between animals was much greater than we were accustomed to in our previous work with isolated hepatocytes and plasma membrane preparations. The thin-layer chromatographic assays for DAG and PA, as useful as they had been, were not precise enough for the *in vivo* work. For DAG the DAG kinase assay offered superior precision (22); for PA we devised a new assay that was far more reproducible and sensitive than previous methods (49). PA was first separated from lyso-PA on silicic acid mini-columns, then deacylated by the gentle procedure, using methylamine as described by Clarke and Dawson (50). The glycerol phosphate formed was then assayed using glycerol phosphate dehydrogenase, and the product, NADH, was measured by HPLC (51). This assay may appear laborious, but we could assay up to 50 extracts in 1 day.

The levels of both DAG and PA were significantly higher in the right lobe of partially hepatectomized rats (Fig. 14) when compared to sham-operated controls (in the two-thirds hepatectomy the left and median lobes are removed) (52). This effect was evidence as early as 30 min after surgery, making it one of the earliest observed. Triglyceride also accumulated in livers from partially hepatectomized rats but not until 8–24 hr (52), when the liver became visibly fatty. The changes in PA and DAG occurred before the large increase in DNA synthesis, which starts at about 12 hr post-

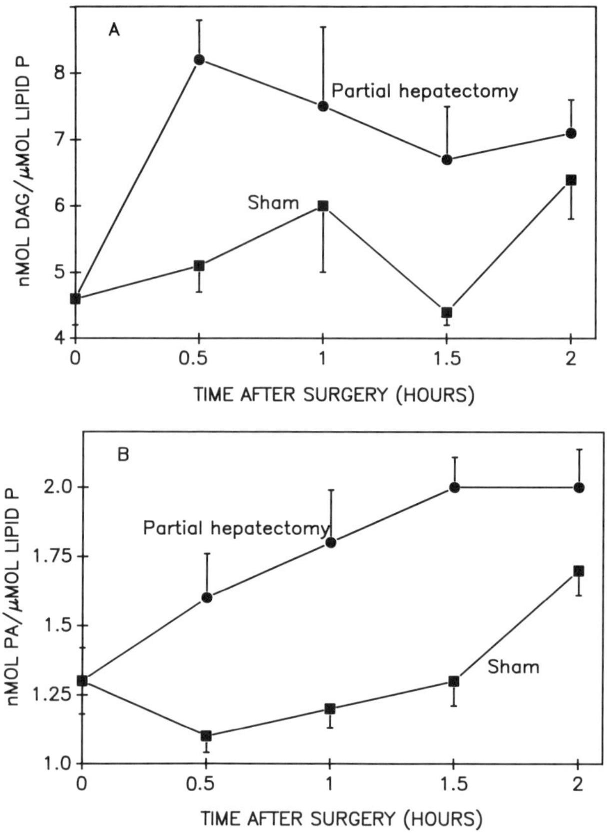

FIGURE 14

Accumulation of (A) diacylglycerol (DAG) and (B) phosphatidate (PA) in the right lobes of livers from partially hepatectomized and sham-operated rats. (From Ref. 52.)

hepatectomy. The hormonal control of liver regeneration has been investigated by many workers, who have determined that norepinephrine (53), vasopressin (54), epidermal growth factor (55), glucagon (56), and insulin (56) are necessary for regeneration. The first three hormones have been shown to elicit PA and DAG in isolated hepatocytes, and glucagon potentiates the actions of norepinephrine and vasopressin (9, 26, 43). Taken together, these facts suggest that these lipids may function in the control of DNA synthesis and mitogenesis.

Both PA and DAG are mitogenic for cultured fibroblasts (45–48). We tested whether PA and DAG caused increased tritiated thymidine incorporation into DNA in isolated hepatocytes cultured under serum-free conditions (57). Neither lipid was effective at concentrations up to 100 μg/ml, under conditions in which norepinephrine stimulated thymidine incorporation 4-fold (unpublished observations; 57). PA was cytotoxic at high concentrations, but bovine serum albumin protected against this toxicity. The negative results seen with PA may be a result of its inability to reach the inner leaflet of the plasma membrane, as reported by Pagano and Longmuir (58). The role of PA and DAG in liver regeneration remains unclear, but we achieved our goal of observing increases in these lipids under physiological conditions.

Role of DAG and PA in Liver Function

The role of sustained increases in DAG due to the breakdown of PC may be the biological counterpart of stimulation of hepatocytes with PMA. In hepatocytes PMA produced decreases in PIP_2 hydrolysis elicited by vasopressin and epinephrine (18, 19), slowly inhibited glycogen synthase (59), and stimulated the Na^+ pump (60). The short-chain DAGs, which have proved so useful in other cell types, are rapidly hydrolyzed by hepatocytes and have not been helpful to us (unpublished observations). One might theorize that the sustained elevation of DAG regulates cellular events with prolonged time courses (e.g., synthesis of organelles and gene regulation). Unfortunately, isolated hepatocytes in suspension have a lifetime of only a few hours, insufficient for this type of investigation. With the exception of the mitogenicity study described above, we have not examined the effects of PMA and DAG on cultured cells, in which the time frame is more appropriate. Consequently, the effects of prolonged elevation of DAG await exploration.

The role of PA is also largely unknown. An oft-reported effect of PA is to elevate $[Ca^{2+}]_i$ (31, 45). We have found that PA supplied "dry" (i.e., oxidized) by the manufacturer can cause mobilization of intracellular Ca^{2+}. Fresh unoxidized PA had no effect on hepatocyte $[Ca^{2+}]_i$ (unpublished observations). It appears that this effect may be due to a product of PA breakdown (e.g., lyso-PA) which mobilizes Ca^{2+} (61), and not to PA itself. We have observed that exogenously added PA lowered the amount of cAMP produced in response to glucagon, through a pertussin toxin-sensitive mechanism (62). This effect of PA has been described in other types of cells, using other agonists, and is apparently mediated by G_i, the guanine nucleotide-binding protein that inhibits adenylate cyclase (31). We have also observed that exogenous PA can activate phosphorylase via a pathway that does not involve increases in $[Ca^{2+}]_i$ or cAMP, the known activators of phosphorylase through phosphorylase kinase (62).

In an attempt to explain the effect of PA on phosphorylase, we have begun to investigate its role in protein phosphorylation. A protein kinase could mediate some of the effects of PA within the cell, similarly to other second messenger systems. Both phosphorylase kinase (63) and PKC (64) are known to be activated by PA. We have observed PA-dependent phosphorylation of certain proteins in rat liver cytosol that are not due to PKC, but this area will remain unclear until the kinase(s) responsible is purified. We are currently attempting this task.

Future Directions

Although we have learned much about PC breakdown in the past few years, much more is unknown. Augert *et al.* (15) recently presented evidence that multiple pools of PC are present in the hepatocyte and that PA and DAG may be formed from separate pools of PC. They labeled isolated hepatocytes with tritiated 1-*O*-alkyl-2-lysoglycero-3-phosphocholine to label the cellular (alkyl) PC. With labeling periods of 5–30 min, vasopressin elicited the accumulation of labeled alkylacylglycerol (the analog of DAG), but not labeled alkyl-PA. Similar findings were observed when radioactive lyso-PC, PC, or phosphatidylethanolamine were used in short-term labeling periods. If tritiated 1-*O*-alkyl-2-lyso-glycero-3-phosphocholine were injected intraportally 20 hr prior to isolation of the hepatocytes, vasopressin could elicit both labeled (alkyl) PA and DAG (15). Thus, it appears that PA and DAG may be formed from separate pools of PC. We are presently investigating the nature and location of these pools.

The Phospholipases C and D that hydrolyze PC appear to be localized to the plasma membrane. PC is present at approximately 18 nmol/mg of wet weight in the hepatocyte (14), but only 1–2% is localized in the plasma membrane. The amounts of PA and DAG that are formed in response to vasopressin at 100 n*M* are roughly equivalent to all of the PC in the plasma membrane. This would not be compatible with life for the cell unless the PC were rapidly reformed or reincorporated into the membrane. To compound matters it is almost certain that PC in only one of the leaflets of the plasma membrane is hydrolyzed. We theorize that DAG and PA are shuttled out of the plasma membrane and that membrane PC is rapidly replenished by some mechanism(s). Pelech and Vance (65) pointed out that the breakdown and resynthesis of PC are part of a cycle; the hormonal regulation of this cycle will engage researchers for some time to come.

References

1. P. F. Blackmore and J. H. Exton, *in* "Methods in Enzymology" (L. Birnbaumer and B. W. O'Malley, eds.), Vol. 109, pp. 550–558. Academic Press, Orlando, Florida, 1985.
2. A. Kishimoto, Y., Takai, T. Mori, U. Kikkawa, and Y. Nishizuka, *J. Biol. Chem.* **255,** 2273–2276 (1980).
3. M. Go, K. Sekiguchi, H. Nomura, U. Kikkawa, and Y. Nishizuka, *Biochem. Biophys. Res. Commun.* **144,** 598–605 (1987).
4. A. A. Abdel-Latif, R. A. Akhtar, and J. N. Hawthorne, *Biochem. J.* **162,** 61–73 (1977).
5. H. Streb, R. F. Irvine, M. J. Berridge, and I. Schultz, *Nature (London)* **306,** 67–69 (1983).
6. M. J. Berridge, *Biochem. J.* **220,** 345–360 (1984).
7. Y. Nishizuka, *Science* **225,** 1365–1370 (1984).
8. J. G. Hamilton and K. Comai, *J. Lipid Res.* **25,** 1142–1148 (1984).
9. S. B. Bocckino, P. F. Blackmore, and J. H. Exton, *J. Biol. Chem.* **260,** 14201–14207 (1985).
10. E. G. Bligh and W. J. Dyer, *Can. J. Biochem. Physiol.* **37,** 911–917 (1959).
11. D. R. Cooper, H. Hernandez, J. Y. Kuo, and R. V. Farese, *Arch. Biochem. Biophys.* **276,** 486–494 (1990).
12. G. Augert, P. F. Blackmore, and J. H. Exton, *J. Biol. Chem.* **264,** 2574–2580 (1989).
13. B. J. Holub and A. Kuksis, *Adv. Lipid Res.* **16,** 1–125 (1978).
14. G. M. Patton, J. M. Fasulo, and S. J. Robins, *J. Lipid Res.* **23,** 190–196 (1982).
15. G. Augert, S. B. Bocckino, P. F. Blackmore, and J. H. Exton, *J. Biol. Chem.* **264,** 21689–21698 (1989).
16. R. A. Mufson, E. Okin, and I. B. Weinstein, *Carcinogenesis* **2,** 1095–1102 (1981).
17. R. I. Grove and S. D. Schimmel, *Biochem. Biophys. Res. Commun.* **102,** 158–164 (1981).
18. C. J. Lynch, R. Charest, S. B. Bocckino, J. H. Exton, and P. F. Blackmore, *J. Biol. Chem.* **260,** 2844–2851 (1985).
19. R. H. Cooper, K. E. Coll, and J. R. Williamson, *J. Biol. Chem.* **260,** 3281–3288 (1985).
20. L. W. Daniel, M. Waite, and R. L. Wykle, *J. Biol. Chem.* **261,** 9128–9132 (1986).
21. J. M. Besterman, V. Duronio, and P. Cuatrecasas, *Proc. Natl. Acad. Sci. U.S.A.* **83,** 6785–6789 (1986).
22. J. Preiss, C. R. Loomis, W. R. Bishop, R. Stein, J. E. Niedel, and R. M. Bell, *J. Biol. Chem.* **261,** 8597–8600 (1986).
23. H. R. Irving and J. H. Exton, *J. Biol. Chem.* **262,** 3440–3443 (1987).
24. M. Hokin-Neaverson, *Biochem. Biophys. Res. Commun.* **58,** 763–768 (1974).
25. S. Cockcroft, *Biochim. Biophys. Acta* **795,** 37–46 (1984).
26. S. B. Bocckino, P. F. Blackmore, P. B. Wilson, and J. H. Exton, *J. Biol. Chem.* **262,** 15309–15315 (1987).
27. K. Nakamura and S. Handa, *Anal. Biochem.* **142,** 406–410 (1984).
28. W. R. Bishop, B. R. Ganong, and R. M. Bell, *J. Biol. Chem.* **261,** 6993–7000 (1986).
29. D. de Chaffoy de Courcelles, P. Roevens, and H. Van Belle, *J. Biol. Chem.* **260,** 15762–15770 (1985).
30. M. M. Billah, S. Eckel, T. J. Mullmann, R. W. Egan, and M. I. Siegel, *J. Biol. Chem.* **264,** 17069–17077 (1989).
31. T. Murayama and M. Ui, *J. Biol. Chem.* **262,** 5522–5529 (1987).
32. T. M. Wright, L. A. Rangan, H. S. Shih, and D. M. Raben, *J. Biol. Chem.* **263,** 9374–9380 (1988).
33. R. J. Uhing, V. Prpic, H. Jiang, and J. H. Exton, *J. Biol. Chem.* **261,** 2140–2146 (1986).
34. T. Taki and J. N. Kanfer, *J. Biol. Chem.* **254,** 9761–9765 (1979).
35. P. G. Roughan and C. R. Slack, *Biochim. Biophys. Acta* **431,** 86–95 (1976).

36. R. M. C. Dawson, *Biochem. J.* **102,** 205–210 (1967).
37. S. B. Bocckino, P. B. Wilson, and J. H. Exton, *FEBS Lett.* **225,** 201–207 (1987).
38. S. A. Wrighton, J.-K. Pai, and G. C. Mueller, *Carcinogenesis* **4,** 1247–1251 (1983).
39. G. C. Mueller, M. F. Fleming, M. A. LeMahieu, G. S. Lybrand, and K. J. Barry, *Proc. Natl. Acad. Sci. U.S.A.* **85,** 9778 –9782 (1988).
40. R. Chalifour and J. N. Kanfer, *J. Neurochem.* **39,** 299–305 (1982).
41. C. J. Lynch, P. F. Blackmore, R. Charest, and J. H. Exton, *Mol. Pharmacol.* **28,** 93–99 (1985).
42. F. L. Dunn, T. J. Brennan, A. E. Nelson, and G. L. Robertson, *J. Clin. Invest.* **52,** 3212–3219 (1973).
43. N. G. Morgan, R. Charest, P. F. Blackmore, and J. H. Exton, *Proc. Natl. Acad. Sci. U.S.A.* **81,** 4208–4212 (1984).
44. G. M. Higgins and R. M. Anderson, *Arch. Pathol.* **12,** 186–202 (1931).
45. W. H. Moolenaar, W. Kruijer, B. C. Tilly, I. Verlaan, A. J. Bierman, and S. W. de Laat, *Nature (London)* **323,** 171–173 (1986).
46. D. W. Siegmann, *Biochem. Biophys. Res. Commun.* **145,** 228–233 (1987).
47. C.-L. Yu, M.-H. Tsai, and D. W. Stacey, *Cell* **52,** 63–71 (1988).
48. E. Rozengurt, A. Rodriguez-Pena, M. Coombs, and J. Sinnett-Smith, *Proc. Natl. Acad. Sci. U.S.A.* **81,** 5748–5752 (1984).
49. S. B. Bocckino, P. Wilson, and J. H. Exton, *Anal. Biochem.* **180,** 24–27 (1989).
50. N. G. Clarke and R. M. C. Dawson, *Biochem. J.* **195,** 301–306 (1981).
51. T. F. Kalhorn, K. E. Thummel, S. D. Nelson, and J. T. Slattery, *Anal. Biochem.* **151,** 343–347 (1985).
52. S. B. Bocckino, P. B. Wilson, and J. H. Exton, *Biochem. Biophys. Res. Commun.* **104,** 290–294 (1989).
53. J. L. Cruise, S. J. Knechtle, R. R. Bollinger, C. Kuhn, and G. Michalopoulos, *Hepatology* **7,** 1189–1194 (1987).
54. W. E. Russell and N. L. Bucher, *Am. J. Physiol.* **245,** G321–G324 (1983).
55. P. S. Olsen, S. Boesby, P. Kirkegaard, K. Therkelson, T. Almdal, S. S. Paulsen, and E. Nexo, *Hepatology* **8,** 992–996 (1988).
56. N. L. Bucher and M. N. Swaffield, *Proc. Natl. Acad. Sci. U.S.A.* **72,** 1157–1160 (1975).
57. J. L. Cruise, K. A. Houck, and G. Michalopoulos, *Science* **227,** 749–751 (1985).
58. R. E. Pagano and K. J. Longmuir, *J. Biol. Chem.* **260,** 1909–1916 (1985).
59. P. F. Blackmore, W. G. Strickland, S. B. Bocckino, and J. H. Exton, *Biochem. J.* **237,** 235–242 (1986).
60. C. J. Lynch, P. B. Wilson, P. F. Blackmore, and J. H. Exton, *J. Biol. Chem.* **261,** 14551–14556 (1986).
61. K. Jalink, E. J. van Corven, and W. H. Moolenaar, *J. Biol. Chem.* **265,** 12232–12239 (1990).
62. S. B. Bocckino, P. F. Blackmore, and J. H. Exton, *FASEB J.* **2,** A1367 (1988).
63. A. I. Negami, H. Sasaki, and H. Yamamura, *Biochem. Biophys. Res. Commun.* **131,** 712–719 (1985).
64. K. Kaibuchi, Y. Takai, and Y. Nishizuka, *J. Biol. Chem.* **256,** 7146–7149 (1981).
65. S. L. Pelech and D. E. Vance, *Trends Biochem. Sci.* **14,** 28–30 (1989).

CHAPTER 5

Calcium Translocation in Signal Transduction

Christian Van Delden, Marisa E. E. Jaconi, Didier Pittet, Nicolas Demaurex, Karl-Heinz Krause, and Daniel P. Lew

Infectious Diseases Division
Geneva University Hospital
1211 Geneva, Switzerland

Introduction

Neutrophils are vital for human defense not only against bacteria and fungi, but they also play an important role against viruses and protozoa (1, 2). Neutrophils are among the most motile mammalian cells, continuously leaving the vascular compartment and crawling into tissues in search of invading microorganisms. When they encounter such targets, which they recognize through specific cell surface receptors, signal transduction occurs, leading to a variety of biological responses. These include adherence, directional movement (chemotaxis), engulfment (phagocytosis), and secretion of granule contents (exocytosis), as well as generation of highly reactive oxygen metabolites at the level of the plasma membrane (the respiratory burst). The integrity and sequence of all these events are essential for the broad antimicrobial activity of these cells, as clearly dem-

Cellular and Molecular Mechanisms of Inflammation, Volume 3

onstrated by the recurrent infections observed in patients with specific genetic defects in any of these steps (3).

Early in the 1980s it was discovered that a large variety of receptors for hormones, neurotransmitters, and, more specifically, several types of receptors in neutrophils are coupled via a family of nucleotide (GTP)-binding proteins to a plasma membrane phospholipase C (4). Phospholipase C cleaves phosphatidylinositol bisphosphate ($PtInsP_2$) into inositol trisphosphate [$Ins(1,4,5)P_3$] and diacylglycerol (DAG). The two latter compounds act as intracellular messengers which mobilize calcium from intracellular stores and activate protein kinase C, respectively.

In more recent years the wealth of discovery in the field is such that only some—arbitrarily chosen—major reviews and key articles can be cited here. Important advances in this field have indicated the following:

1. The inositol phosphate pathway [including its regulation and subcellular localization (5–11)] is increasingly complex. A specific membrane-bound phosphatase and a specific soluble kinase generate, respectively, $InsP_2$ and $Ins(1,3,4,5)P_4$, from $Ins(1,4,5)P_3$, and there is production of highly phosphorylated inositol phosphates (there are several $InsP_4$, $InsP_5$, and $InsP_6$). Additional information has been provided on the metabolism, regulation, and role of the phosphoinositol pathway, the source of different inositol phosphates. In particular more is known about the regulation of the kinases generating PtIns, PtInsP, and $PtInsP_2$, and $PtInsP_3$.

2. A variety of G regulatory proteins have been characterized, purified, and cloned in many cellular systems, including phagocytic cells (12–16). Multiple functions have been attributed to these proteins, including coupling of receptors to their catalytic unit (e.g., phospholipase C, adenylate cyclase, and guanylate cyclase), regulation of plasma membrane channels, enzymes (e.g., cGMP phosphodiesterase), and even possibly the control of exocytosis and oxidative burst activity.

3. The regulation and role of $[Ca^{2+}]_i$ have been examined. Considerable controversy still surrounds the nature of the intracellular stores that, in myeloid cells, have been defined as calciosomes (17–19). Important questions include: Are calciosomes discrete entities, or linked to the endoplasmic reticulum (ER)? Are there one, two, or even more intracellular Ca^{2+}stores, and how many of them are $Ins(1,4,5)P_3$ sensitive? Even more confusing is the area dealing with mechanisms of Ca^{2+} influx across the plasma membrane [see recent reviews on Ca^{2+} influx, the role of $Ins(1,3,4,5)P_4$, and the quantal model proposed by Irvine and colleagues (20–22)]. Increasingly sophisticated equipment and the development of new fluorescent probes allowed the detection of subcellular $[Ca^{2+}]_i$ gra-

dients and the observation that $[Ca^{2+}]_i$ appears to oscillate in several cellular systems, including neutrophils (23–25). It has also been established more solidly that Ca^{2+} plays a key role in the control of certain cell functions (e.g., exocytosis). However, additional signals must be important in handling multiple other cellular processes (e.g., locomotion and intracellular traffic of organelles).

4. Phospholipid metabolism and cellular activation have been investigated. It has become clear that many of the receptors capable of stimulating $PtInsP_2$ breakdown also stimulate the breakdown of phosphatidylcholine (PC) (26–29). The hydrolysis of PC by phospholipase A_2 (PLA_2) is an important source of arachidonic acid, which is subsequently metabolized to a variety of functionally significant eicosanoids. PC can also be hydrolyzed by phospholipases C and D to yield DAG and phosphatidic acid (PA). In fact, this last pathway is probably the most important quantitative source of DAG during cell stimulation (11).

5. It has been realized that protein kinase C is a family of enzymes with regions of homology, but also clearly distinct domains and enzymological properties. Members of this family are differently distributed in various cell types. The enzyme appears to interact with many signaling pathways and display functions in the processing and modulation of cellular responses to external stimuli (30–32).

6. Additional signals have been studied. The existence in phagocytes of excitatory signals in addition to Ca^{2+} and protein kinase C, particularly in activation of the oxidase, has been suggested by several workers, including Rossi and co-workers (33), Grinstein and Furuya (34), Korchak *et al.* (35), and Dewald *et al.* (36). Potential candidates for such activation signals include products generated by PLD, PLA_2, or various protein kinases, including tyrosine kinases and phosphoprotein phosphatases.

7. In neutrophils studies have been carried out characterizing various protein kinases, such as isoenzymes of protein kinase C, cAMP-dependent protein kinases, Ca^{2+}-calmodulin-dependent protein kinases, tyrosine kinase S, and histone 144 kinase (37–39).

8. Control of cytoplasmic actin has been the subject of study as well. Several workers on phagocyte physiology have also provided clues as to how cells control cytoplasmic actin assembly. Interaction of receptors coupled to G regulatory proteins to the actin network has been demonstrated (40, 41). One of the most intriguing recent discoveries is a potential role of $PtInsP_2$ as an inhibitor of interaction of actin with actin regulatory factors [e.g., profilin or gelsolin (42)].

This review focuses on our mayor area of interest: the regulation and role of $[Ca^{2+}]_i$ in neutrophil activation.

Ca^{2+} Signal: Studies in Cell Populations and Single Neutrophils

The introduction of fluorescent indicators of $[Ca^{2+}]_i$ (e.g., quin2 and fura-2) enabled the analysis of $[Ca^{2+}]_i$ transients during neutrophil activation. Studies in populations of neutrophils (3) showed an average resting $[Ca^{2+}]_i$ of ~100 n*M*. In response to stimulation with f–Met–Leu–Phe (fMLP, a synthetic formyl peptide that resembles products of bacterial metabolism), $[Ca^{2+}]_i$ increases to micromolar concentrations and returns to baseline within approximately 10 min. This $[Ca^{2+}]_i$ increase is partially dependent on extracellular Ca^{2+}; that is, the initial rate of the $[Ca^{2+}]_i$ increase is unchanged in a Ca^{2+}-free solution, while the prolonged period of the $[Ca^{2+}]_i$ increase is abolished under these conditions (43–45). These results led to the conclusion that the $[Ca^{2+}]_i$ increase in response to chemoattractants consists of two components, an initial release of Ca^{2+} from an intracellular storage site, and a more delayed influx of Ca^{2+} across the plasma membrane. The Ca^{2+} ionophore ionomycin is able to induce $[Ca^{2+}]_i$ increases in the absence of extracellular Ca^{2+}, as is seen for fMLP stimulation, suggesting that the intracellular Ca^{2+} storage site is a vesicular organelle (43).

The use of new highly fluorescent intracellular calcium indicators (23, 25) such as fura-2 has allowed monitoring of $[Ca^{2+}]_i$ at the single-cell level in a variety of cellular systems, including neutrophils. Initial studies in single adherent neutrophils using either quin2 or fura-2 showed the presence of single $[Ca^{2+}]_i$ transients concomitant with the initial step of adherence to glass slides (46). These studies also suggested the presence of subcellular $[Ca^{2+}]_i$ gradients upon cellular movement (47). Measurements of single-cell $[Ca^{2+}]_i$ during phagocytosis of C3bi-opsonized yeast particles were performed and a rapid rise in $[Ca^{2+}]_i$ (followed by one or more $[Ca^{2+}]_i$ peaks) was observed during contact with the particle (48). These results suggest a role of $[Ca^{2+}]_i$ in some of the events associated with phagocytosis (see "Plasma Membrane Ca^{2+} Pump").

We have studied $[Ca^{2+}]_i$ in single neutrophils adherent to fibronectin- or albumin-coated surfaces. While neutrophils in suspension maintain stable $[Ca^{2+}]_i$ basal levels, we observed spontaneous oscillations of $[Ca^{2+}]_i$ (49), with an average peak amplitude of 80 n*M* and a mean duration of 30 sec. This spontaneous $[Ca^{2+}]_i$ activity may be dissociated from the $[Ca^{2+}]_i$ activity triggered by chemoattractant receptor stimulation. Activation of neutrophils by the chemoattractant fMLP at low concentrations (10^{-10} *M*) triggers sustained $[Ca^{2+}]_i$ oscillations, whereas continuous $[Ca^{2+}]_i$ rises were observed at high agonist concentrations (10^{-6} *M*). This study raised the interesting possibility that certain neutrophil functions might be controlled by $[Ca^{2+}]_i$ oscillations, rather than by sustained alterations of $[Ca^{2+}]_i$. Stimulation of various other cell types with Ins(1,4,5)P_3-generating agonists has similarly been shown to induce oscillating elevations of $[Ca^{2+}]_i$ (17). In neutrophils and other nonexcitable cells $[Ca^{2+}]_i$ oscillations seem to be due to the intermittent release of Ca^{2+} from intracellular stores, rather than to intermittent Ca^{2+} influx (17, 49). It has been proposed that this type of $[Ca^{2+}]_i$ oscillation is due to intermittent generation of Ins(1,4,5)P_3 (50). However, intracellular application of nonhydrolyzable InsP_3 analogs by microinjection or microperfusion also induces oscillating elevations of $[Ca^{2+}]_i$ in various cell types (51, 52). Thus, the mechanism of the oscillating Ca^{2+} release might be distal to Ins(1,4,5)P_3 generation.

At least two subcellular organelles play a crucial role in Ca^{2+} homeostasis in myeloid cells: the plasma membrane and an Ins(1,4,5)P_3-sensitive intracellular Ca^{2+} store, the calciosome.

Neutrophil Plasma Membrane: Ion Channels, Membrane Potential, and Ca^{2+} Influx

Plasma membrane ion channels play an important role in the regulation of cellular activity and as effector proteins for many cellular functions. Despite substantial progress in the understanding of signal transduction and cellular activation in neutrophils, little is known about the nature and properties of ion channels in these cells. As observed in most other cell types, the intracellular concentrations of various ions are different from those observed in the extracellular medium. Intracellular ion concentrations are high for K^+, low for Na^+, and extremely low for Ca^{2+} (43, 53). The intracellular Cl^- concentration in human neutrophils is ~80 m*M* (53), thus lower than that for extracellular Cl^- (140 m*M*), but relatively high compared to those of other cells. Ionic gradients, like those observed in neutrophils, are determined by the transport proteins in the cell membrane, including pumps, transporters, and channels. Pumps use cellular sources of energy (e.g., ATP) to transport ions against electrochemical gradients. Other membrane transporters perform ion exchange, cotransport, and countertransport to move ions across membranes. Their capacity is relatively low (maximum of 10^3 ions per second). Channels, in contrast, are pores that allow passive movement of ions down favorable electrochemical gradients. They can be in an open (i.e., active) or closed state. Channels are often ion selective and thus provide a means for making the plasma membrane conductive for specific ions. When compared to other transport proteins, ion channels have a very high capacity (at least 10^6 ions per second).

Channels have a variety of functions in different cell types. Most cells have K^+ channels that are active in the resting cell and lead to K^+ efflux because of the gradient between the high intracellular and low extracellular K^+ concentrations. If the cell membrane is relatively impermeant for other ions, K^+ efflux cannot be counterbalanced and leads to build-up of a negative charge in the cell interior (i.e., a negative resting potential). In so-called excitable tissues (e.g., nerve and muscle) stimulation of cells opens Na^+ channels; Na^+ influx depolarizes the cell and leads to an action potential. A variety of cells have different types of Ca^{2+} channels that allow Ca^{2+} influx and an increase in the cytosolic free Ca^{2+} concentration during cellular activation. Many cells have Cl^- channels which may be involved in the regulation of membrane potential (e.g., GABA receptor in the brain), fluid secretion (epithelial cells), or cellular volume homeostasis (54–56).

Plasma membrane channels of small cells (e.g., neutrophils) can be studied by indirect methods or directly by the patch–clamp technique. The indirect methods include radioactive tracer fluxes, determination of intracellular ion concentrations with fluorescent dyes, or measurement of plasma membrane potential with charged lipophilic compounds. The three indirect methods, however, give only limited information about the ion channels of a cell. Using radioactive tracer fluxes, it is difficult to distinguish between transport processes and conductive pathways. Changes in intracellular ion concentrations are the net result of the activity of all the different transport and conductive pathways for a certain ion. Plasma membrane potential reflects the sum of all electrogenic processes across the plasma membrane. The patch–clamp method, in contrast, allows direct determination of plasma membrane ionic conductances and the study of their regulation.

We now review recent data on the electrophysiological properties of human neutrophils and the interaction of ion channels with the Ca^{2+} messenger system.

Studies of Membrane Potential in Neutrophils

Using membrane potential-sensitive fluorescent dyes or radiotracers, the membrane potential in populations of neutrophils has been studied. Efforts have been made to determine the resting potential, the potential changes during cellular activation, and the ionic basis of these phenomena.

The resting potential of neutrophils has been estimated to be between

−20 and −105 mV (53, 57–62). These large deviations show that the method is poorly suited for the determination of absolute values. Still, most groups now agree on resting values between −50 and −60 mV. An increase in the extracellular K^+ concentration depolarizes neutrophils (59). This suggests that, similar to other cell types (see "Introduction"), the resting potential in neutrophils is maintained by a K^+ channel.

Membrane potential changes during cellular activation in neutrophils have been described as follows.

1. Neutrophils depolarize in response to receptor agonists (59), but also in response to agonists that bypass the receptor mechanism [e.g., ionomycin (a calcium ionophore) or phorbol myristate acetate (a protein kinase C activator)] (63).
2. Membrane depolarization in response to receptor agonists is inhibited by the preincubation of cells with pertussis toxin (63). This argues against a mechanism of depolarization that is directly linked to the receptor (as it may be in excitable tissues) and suggests mediation by a G protein.
3. The ionic basis of the depolarizing current in neutrophils has not yet been identified. Replacement of extracellular Na^+ by choline does not affect depolarization (58). As choline is a cation that does not usually pass through Na^+-selective channels, this observation indicates that Na^+ channels are not required for depolarization in neutrophils. However, in other cell types nonselective channels that conduct choline have been described, and a role of nonselective channels in neutrophil depolarization has not yet been excluded. In some cell types closing of K^+ channels or opening of Cl^- channels is thought to depolarize the cells (54, 64). These possibilities have not yet been studied in neutrophils. It has also been proposed that the electron transfer from the cytosol to the extracellular space that occurs during the respiratory burst of neutrophils is electrogenic and leads to plasma membrane depolarization (62).

The physiological role of depolarization in neutrophils is different from that in excitable cells. Neither Ca^{2+} influx nor cellular activation is observed after depolarization of neutrophils by high extracellular K^+ or by Na^+/K^+ ionophores such as gramicidin (65, 66). In contrast, if depolarization precedes cellular stimulation by chemoattractants, the increases in cytosolic Ca^{2+} and cellular responses are diminished (66). In recent studies we could demonstrate that depolarizing agents such as gramicidin and ouabain directly interfere with the generation of Ins(1,4,5)P_3 (67). We have therefore proposed a role of depolarization as negative feedback during neutrophil activation. However, studies that directly manipulate the membrane potential without pharmacological intervention will be necessary to definitely demonstrate this model.

Whole-Cell Patch–Clamp Studies in Human Neutrophils

The patch–clamp technique was initially designed as a method to study single ion channels. However, it rapidly emerged as a technique with a variety of applications, such as the measurement of whole-cell currents in small cells, the study of interactions of intracellular messengers with ion channels, and the study of control of secretion (68, 69). The whole-cell patch–clamp technique measures the channel currents from the entire plasma membrane of a single cell, whereas the single-channel patch–clamp technique measures the current in a randomly chosen small piece of membrane. Accordingly, the whole-cell patch–clamp technique, as compared to single-channel measurements, is better suited for the initial study of cells whose set of ion channels is not yet known. We therefore used the whole-cell patch–clamp technique to study transmembrane currents in adherent neutrophils. As the $[Ca^{2+}]_i$ is known to be an important intracellular messenger in neutrophils, we also studied the modification of whole-cell currents by changes in $[Ca^{2+}]_i$. We found voltage-dependent K^+ channels and Ca^{2+}-activated K^+ and Cl^- channels. Some properties of these channels are described below. (If not stated otherwise, the original reference is Ref. 63.)

Voltage-Dependent K^+ Channel

A voltage-activated current was found in unstimulated neutrophils studied with the whole-cell patch–clamp technique. This channel had a threshold of voltage activation of –60 mV. Maximal activation was observed at 90 mV. No time-dependent inactivation was found, even at large depolarizing voltages. Tail current analysis under varying ionic conditions suggested that the channel was selective for K^+. The channel current showed inward rectification (i.e., a larger conductance for K^+ influx than for K^+ efflux). The channel was blocked by $BaCl_2$, but not by 5-aminopyridine, a blocker of the depolarization-activated K^+ channel of macrophages.

The properties of the channel suggest that it may determine the resting membrane potential of neutrophils as (1) it is found in unstimulated cells, (2) it is K^+ selective and thus generates a negative plasma membrane potential by electrogenic K^+ efflux, and (3) it has a threshold of voltage activation of –60 mV and therefore hyperpolarizes neutrophils only to this voltage (i.e., the membrane potential of resting neutrophils; a K^+ channel that is independent of voltage would be expected to hyperpolarize cells to −80 mV, the reversal potential of K^+). Given the role of the membrane potential in signal transduction of neutrophils (see the previous section), the regulation of the resting potential by the voltage-dependent K^+ channel might play an important role in determining the sensitivity of neutrophils to chemotactic stimulation. It will therefore be of major interest to study the pharmacology of this channel, as well as its possible regulation by intracellular messengers.

Ca^{2+}-Activated K^+ and Cl^- Channels in Neutrophils

Activation of neutrophils by various receptor agonists leads to an elevation of $[Ca^{2+}]_i$. In other cell types such $[Ca^{2+}]_i$ elevations activate a variety of channels. It was therefore of interest to study the effect of Ca^{2+} on channel currents in neutrophils. We exposed neutrophils in the whole-cell patch configuration to the Ca^{2+} ionophore ionomycin. This procedure led to an increase in whole-cell currents, thus demonstrating the presence of Ca^{2+}-activated ion channels in neutrophils. Analysis of the ionic selectivity of the Ca^{2+}-activated channels revealed the existence of both Cl^- and K^+ channels.

As many K^+ channels are voltage dependent and Ca^{2+} activated, we considered the possibility that the depolarization-activated K^+ conductances and the Ca^{2+}-activated K^+ conductances reflect two modes of activation of the same channel. However, several observations argue against this possibility. The voltage-activated channel appeared to be independent of intracellular Ca^{2+} concentrations, while the Ca^{2+}-activated K^+ channel appeared to be independent of voltage. In addition the two K^+ channels could be distinguished by their conductive properties. The voltage-activated K^+ channel was inwardly rectifying; that is, K^+ passed more readily from the outside of the cell to the inside than from the inside to the outside. The Ca^{2+}-activated K^+ channel, in contrast, was outwardly rectifying.

The effect of a concomitant Ca^{2+}-induced opening of Cl^- and K^+ channels on net salt fluxes in a neutrophil would be a loss of KCl to the extracellular space. Such a loss of intracellular KCl has been shown in other cell types to be accompanied by a loss of intracellular water and a decrease in cell volume (55, 56, 70).

What could be the physiological significance of a Ca^{2+}-induced decrease in cell volume? In other cell types a Ca^{2+}-conductive pathway sensitive to cell volume has been described (55, 56). Exposure of such cells to hypotonic solutions leads to the following cascade of events: an increase in cell volume, activation of volume-sensitive Ca^{2+} influx, activation of Ca^{2+}-gated K^+ and Cl^- channels, a net loss of KCl and water, and a decrease in cell volume toward the normal level. Neutrophils might have such a mechanism, as they are relatively resistant to hypotonic solution: Brief exposure to distilled water, a routine step in neutrophil purification which lyses red blood cells, does not damage neutrophils. However, no volume-sensitive Ca^{2+} influx has yet been described in neutrophils.

Alternatively, changes in cell volume might be a part of the response to the increase in $[Ca^{2+}]_i$ that occurs during cellular activation. Many neutrophil functions that are mediated or accompanied by rises in $[Ca^{2+}]_i$ (e.g., chemotaxis, adherence to surfaces and spreading, pseudopod formation, and phagocytosis) might necessitate changes in cell volume.

Comparison of Membrane Potential and Ion Channels in Macrophages and Neutrophils

Macrophages are cells that share a variety of properties with neutrophils. It is therefore of interest to compare the results of electrophysiological studies in neutrophils with those obtained in macrophages (63, 71). Resting membrane potential of macrophages and neutrophils has been reported to be in a similar range (i.e., −50 to −60 mV). Voltage-dependent K^+ channels in both cell types, macrophages (71) and neutrophils (63), are likely to maintain this resting potential. However, the neutrophil channel shows distinct properties. It differs from the macrophage channel because it does not deactivate with time, it is not inhibited by 4-aminopyridine, and it shows inward rectification.

After stimulation with chemotactic peptides or Ca^{2+} ionophores, neutrophils depolarize, while macrophages hyperpolarize. Two types of Ca^{2+}-activated K^+ channels have been described in macrophages: a voltage-dependent type and a voltage-independent type. A $[Ca^{2+}]_i$ increase in macrophages should activate these two channels and thereby lead to hyperpolarization. In addition, macrophages possess a hyperpolarization-activated K^+ channel, which might provide further positive feedback to the Ca^{2+}-induced hyperpolarization. Neutrophils have only one kind of Ca^{2+}-activated K^+ channel and no hyperpolarization-activated K^+ channel. However, they have a Ca^{2+}-activated Cl^- channel that has not been described in macrophages. Could this Ca^{2+}-activated Cl^- channel play a role in the depolarization produced during neutrophil activation? The intracellular Cl^- concentration in neutrophils is relatively high (53). The reversal potential for Cl^- is therefore less negative than the resting plasma membrane potential (i.e., −14 versus −60 mV). Activation of Cl^- channels by Ca^{2+} could therefore depolarize neutrophils, depending on the relative contribution of Ca^{2+}-activated Cl^- channels and Ca^{2+}-activated K^+ channels. However, depolarization of neutrophils in response to physiological stimuli is only partially Ca^{2+} dependent, and Ca^{2+}-independent depolarization is observed in response to phorbol esters. Thus, while Ca^{2+} activation of Cl^- channels might contribute to depolarization in neutrophils, it is unlikely to be the only mechanism.

Plasma Membrane Ca^{2+} Channels and Ca^{2+} Influx

No structural information is available on the plasma membrane Ca^{2+} channels of neutrophils or related cells. In patch–clamp studies in neutrophils, a Ca^{2+}-activated nonspecific cation channel able to conduct Ca^{2+} has been observed (72, 73). However, so far no evidence is available for a physiological role of this channel in stimulated Ca^{2+} influx in neutrophils. Similarly, there are no convincing direct electrophysiological measurements of Ca^{2+} influx in most other nonexcitable cells. However, Ca^{2+} influx in response to receptor activation can be demonstrated clearly in studies with Ca^{2+}-sensitive fluorescent dyes. The molecular mechanism of the receptor-operated Ca^{2+} influx in neutrophils is not yet understood. It can be distinguished from Ca^{2+} influx through voltage-gated Ca^{2+} channels in excitable tissues by the following criteria: (1) It cannot be elicited by plasma membrane depolarization (65), (2) it is increased by hyperpolarization during receptor activation (66), and (3) it is not inhibited by blockers of voltage-gated Ca^{2+} channels (e.g., 1,4-dihydropyridines) (65).

Intracellular application of Ins(1,4,5)P_3 by microinjection or microperfusion has not yet been performed in neutrophils, but has been shown to induce Ca^{2+} influx in various types of nonexcitable cells. Three explanations have been proposed to account for these results.

1. The plasma membrane might have Ins(1,4,5)P_3-sensitive Ca^{2+} channels. Patch–clamp studies in lymphocytes favor this theory (74).
2. A metabolite of Ins(1,4,5)P_3, particularly inositol 1,3,4,5-tetrakisphosphate [Ins(1,3,4,5)P_4], might be the intracellular mediator of Ca^{2+} influx. In one study concomitant microperfusion of Ins(1,3,4,5)P_4 potentiated the Ins(1,4,5)P_3 effect on Ca^{2+} influx (21). We have monitored in parallel Ca^{2+}influx and inositol phosphate levels in populations of HL-60 cells. These studies revealed a good temporal correlation between Ca^{2+} influx and Ins(1,3,4,5)P_4 levels, but not with the level of any other inositol phosphate (75). However, in other cell types nonmetabolizable Ins(1,4,5)P_3 analogs induce Ca^{2+} influx (76).
3. The filling state of the intracellular Ca^{2+} pool regulates Ca^{2+} influx (i.e., capacitative Ca^{2+} entry). Thus, Ins(1,4,5)P_3 would regulate Ca^{2+} influx indirectly by its effect on the filling state of the intracellular Ca^{2+} pool. This theory is supported by studies that demonstrate that Thapsigargin, a com-

pound that empties the Ins(1,4,5)P_3-sensitive Ca^{2+} pool by inhibition of Ca^{2+} uptake, also induces Ca^{2+} influx (77, 78).

Plasma Membrane Ca^{2+} Pump

The plasma membrane Ca^{2+} pump, present in virtually all cell types, was originally characterized in red blood cells. Our present knowledge of the plasma membrane pump of neutrophils is based on studies of inside-out plasma membrane vesicles (79, 80). The enzyme seems to be, similar to the intracellular Ca^{2+} pump, a Ca^{2+}-ATPase, requiring ATP hydrolysis for activity. However, unlike the intracellular Ca^{2+}-ATPase, the plasma membrane Ca^{2+} pump shares several properties with the erythrocyte-type Ca^{2+}-ATPase: (1) Ca^{2+} uptake is inhibited by low concentrations of vanadate (30 μ*M*), (2) Ca^{2+} uptake is inhibited by calmodulin inhibitors, and (3) addition of exogenous calmodulin increases Ca^{2+} pumping. Recently, a plasma membrane Ca^{2+}-ATPase from human teratoma cells has been cloned (81). Supporting the functional data in neutrophils and other cell types, a calmodulin binding site was demonstrated. The plasma membrane Ca^{2+} pump of neutrophils can be activated by phorbol esters (82), suggesting that this protein is, directly or indirectly, regulated by protein kinase C in addition to its Ca^{2+}/calmodulin regulation. There is no evidence for the involvement of a Na^+/Ca^{2+} exchanger in Ca^{2+} transport to the extracellular space in neutrophils.

Intracellular Ca^{2+} Stores in Myeloid Cells

Ins(1,4,5)P_3-Sensitive Ca^{2+} Stores (Calciosomes)

The identity of the Ins(1,4,5)P_3-sensitive Ca^{2+} store is still a matter of debate. In some nonmuscle cells the organelle specifically devoted to the rapid ATP-dependent uptake of Ca^{2+} and to its release in response to receptor-triggered generation of Ins(1,4,5)P_3 is thought to be the ER. However, results in other cellular systems, including neutrophils and HL-60 cells, suggest the existence of a specialized subcellular structure: the calciosome. By using calcium-selective electrodes and various fractionation procedures, we could study the control of $[Ca^{2+}]_i$ by subcellular structures in neutrophils and HL-60 cells (83).

HL-60 cell homogenates were separated by a discontinuous Percoll gradient. The gradient yielded three fractions. Table I shows the distribution of various marker enzymes (alkaline phosphatase and cholesterol for the plasma membrane, sulfatase C and NADPH–cytochrome *c* reductase for the ER, galactosyltransferase for the Golgi apparatus, and β-glucuronidase for granules) in the three fractions. About 35% of the recovered plasma membrane content was localized in the light-density fraction 3 (F_3). To shift the distribution of plasma membrane toward fractions of higher density, HL-60 cell homogenates were preincubated with digitonin before separation by the gradient. Digitonin is known to bind specifically to the cholesterol-containing plasma membranes and has been used to increase the density of plasma membrane vesicles, which are thereafter shifted toward fractions of higher densities in density gradients (84, 85). Table I

TABLE I

Digitonin-Induced Shift of Organelles in HL-60 Cell Subcellular Fractions[a]

	Digitonin				
Marker enzyme	0 μM	30 μM	50 μM	100 μM	Fraction
Alkaline phosphatase	10 ± 1	11 ± 2	10 ± 1	8 ± 1	F_1
(n = 6)	55 ± 2	59 ± 2	64 ± 1	74 ± 1	F_2
	36 ± 1	31 ± 1	29 ± 2	19 ± 1	F_3
Cholesterol (n = 3)	15 ± 2	ND	4 ± 1	8 ± 2	F_1
	53 ± 4	ND	66 ± 3	72 ± 3	F_2
	35 ± 1	ND	31 ± 3	18 ± 3	F_3
Sulfatase C (n = 5–7)	5 ± 1	4 ± 1[b]	6 ± 1	5 ± 1	F_1
	76 ± 2	77 ± 1[b]	75 ± 2	77 ± 2	F_2
	15 ± 1	20 ± 1[b]	17 ± 1	17 ± 1	F_3
NADPH–Cytochrome	14 ± 5	ND	ND	10 ± 4	F_1
c reductase (n = 3)	65 ± 1	ND	ND	66 ± 3	F_2
	21 ± 5	ND	ND	23 ± 3	F_3
Galactosyltransferase	2 ± 1	1 ± 1[b]	2 ± 1	2 ± 1	F_1
(n = 5)	66 ± 4	60 ± 17[b]	72 ± 6	73 ± 3	F_2
	32 ± 4	39 ± 17[b]	31 ± 6	26 ± 3	F_3
β-Glucuronidase	7 ± 1	9 ± 2[b]	10 ± 1	10 ± 1	F_1
(n = 4)	76 ± 3	76 ± 2[b]	76 ± 1	79 ± 1	F_2
	16 ± 3	15 ± 2[b]	13 ± 2	12 ± 1	F_3

[a]HL-60 cell homogenates were incubated for 10 min at 37°C in the absence or presence of digitonin (30, 50, and 100 μM). Three subcellular fractions (F_1, F_2, and F_3) were obtained by density gradient centrifugation of homogenates. Activities of the various marker enzymes (alkaline phosphatase for the plasma membrane, sulfatase C and NADPH–cytochrome c reductase for the endoplasmic reticulum, β-glucuronidase for granules, and galactosyltransferase for the Golgi apparatus) are expressed as percentages of gradient distribution; that is, the total marker enzyme content of all three subcellular fractions is taken as 100%.

shows the shift of plasma membrane markers toward fractions of higher densities after incubation with increasing concentrations of digitonin. Neither the ER nor the Golgi apparatus nor granule markers showed a significant shift, as expected by their lower cholesterol content. At a digitonin concentration of 100 μM, the plasma membrane content of F_3 was reduced by nearly 50%. Under identical conditions Ca^{2+} uptake and Ins(1,4,5)P_3-induced Ca^{2+} release were predominantly recovered in the light-density F_3. Both parameters were not affected by the digitonin preincubation and were not shifted toward fractions of higher densities when homogenates were preincubated in the presence of digitonin (Fig. 1), indicating that the Ins(1,4,5)P_3-sensitive Ca^{2+} store is an organelle with a low cholesterol content and is not contained in the plasma membrane.

The subcellular distribution of both Ca^{2+} uptake and Ins(1,4,5)P_3-induced Ca^{2+} release did not correlate with the subcellular distribution of the ER markers. Indeed, both markers of the Ins(1,4,5)P_3-sensitive Ca^{2+} store were substantially enriched in the light-density F_3 (Fig. 1), in contrast to markers of the ER (e.g., sulfatase C and NADPH–cytochrome *c* reductase), which were predominantly recovered in the intermediate-density F_2.

We thus could demonstrate that markers for the Ins(1,4,5)P_3-sensitive Ca^{2+} store can be dissociated from markers of plasma membrane and ER and are present in a light density fraction. A further separation from

FIGURE 1

Ca^{2+} uptake and Ins(1,4,5)P_3-induced Ca^{2+} release in HL-60 cell subcellular fractions. HL-60 cells were homogenized by nitrogen cavitation. Three subcellular fractions (F_1, F_2, and F_3) were obtained by density gradient centrifugation of homogenates (H) previously preincubated in the absence [(A) trace a, (B and C) solid bars] or presence of digitonin (100 μM) [(A) trace b, (B and C) stippled bars]. Homogenates and subcellular fractions (0.8 mg of protein in 0.6 ml) were incubated at 37°C, and ambient free Ca^{2+} levels were assessed by the fluorescence of fura-2. (A) Ambient free Ca^{2+}concentrations were monitored in the presence of light-density subcellular fractions (F_3). Ins(1,4,5)P_3 (1 μM) was added where indicated. Traces are from a typical experiment which was repeated four times. (B) Specific Ca^{2+} uptake activity is shown as nanomoles of Ca^{2+} per milligram per minute removed from the medium by intracellular organelles. (C) Specific Ins(1,4,5)P_3-induced Ca^{2+} release activity (nanomoles of Ca^{2+} per milligram of protein) was determined in homogenates and subcellular fractions, using a maximally Ca^{2+}-releasing Ins(1,4,5)P_3 concentration (1 μM) added to the samples once they had reached a steady state of ambient free Ca^{2+} for at least 3 min. Values are means ± SE in n = 4–8 (B) and n = 4 (C) separate experiments.

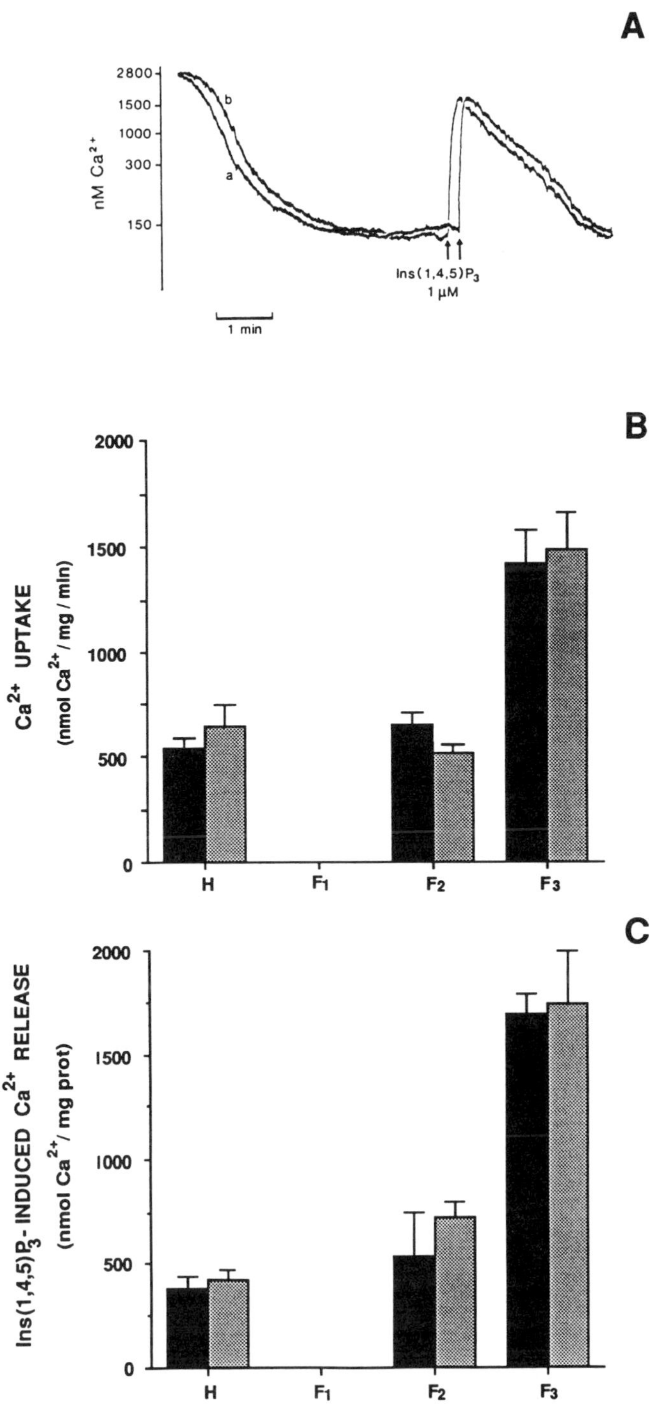
A
nM Ca2+
2800
1500
1000
300
150
b
a
Ins(1,4,5)P3
1 μM
1 min
B
Ca2+ UPTAKE
(nmol Ca2+/ mg / min)
2000
1500
1000
500
0
H
F1
F2
F3
C
Ins(1,4,5)P3- INDUCED Ca2+ RELEASE
(nmol Ca2+/ mg prot)
2000
1500
1000
500
0
H
F1
F2
F3

contaminating endosomes could be achieved by free-flow electrophoresis (83).

Analysis of the fractions described above by staining of sodium dodecyl sulfate (SDS) gels and by $^{45}Ca^{2+}$ overlay of nitrocellulose transfers of SDS gels revealed the presence of a 60-kDa Ca^{2+}-binding protein that copurified with the markers of the Ins(1,4,5)P_3-sensitive Ca^{2+} stores (calreticulin; see "Intravesicular Ca^{2+} Storage Proteins").

These results led to the conclusion that HL-60 cells contain a specialized intracellular compartment involved in Ca^{2+} storage and Ins(1,4,5)P_3-induced Ca^{2+} release. We have proposed to call this compartment the calciosome (Fig. 2).

InsP_3-Insensitive Ca^{2+} Stores

Studies from various laboratories have suggested that there might be intracellular Ca^{2+} stores that are not sensitive to Ins(1,4,5)P_3 (86, 87). Ca^{2+} release from these stores can be pharmacologically induced by caffeine. These stores might physiologically release Ca^{2+} in response to increases of $[Ca^{2+}]_i$ (i.e., Ca^{2+}-induced Ca^{2+} release), but the existence of such additional stores has not yet been demonstrated in neutrophils.

Intracellular Ca^{2+} Pumps (Ca^{2+}-ATPase)

At least three types of intracellular Ca^{2+}-ATPases exist. All of them show a molecular mass of approximately 100 kDa and are structurally distinct from the plasma membrane Ca^{2+}-ATPase. The fast-type Ca^{2+}-ATPase is found exclusively in fast-type skeletal muscle. The slow-type Ca^{2+}-ATPase is found in slow-type skeletal muscle and cardiac muscle. A nonmuscle Ca^{2+}-ATPase is found in a variety of nonmuscle cells. While a separate gene codes for the fast-type ATPase, the latter two types of intracellular Ca^{2+}-ATPases are generated by alternative splicing of the same gene (88, 89).

Another type of intracellular Ca^{2+}-ATPase has been suggested recently. This Ca^{2+}-ATPase would have a molecular mass of 120 kDa and would show a subcellular distribution similar to that of the Ins(1,4,5)P_3-sensitive Ca^{2+} pool (90). In lacrimal acinar cells Ca^{2+} uptake into the InsP_3-sensitive Ca^{2+} pool has been proposed to occur through a mechanism that is energized by a proton gradient (86).

Functional studies in permeabilized neutrophils and neutrophil homogenates (91, 92) demonstrate that the Ca^{2+} pump of the intracellular Ca^{2+} store is a Ca^{2+}-ATPase, functionally similar to the Ca^{2+}-ATPase of the sarcoplasmic reticulum of muscle cells: (1) Ca^{2+} uptake is ATP dependent;

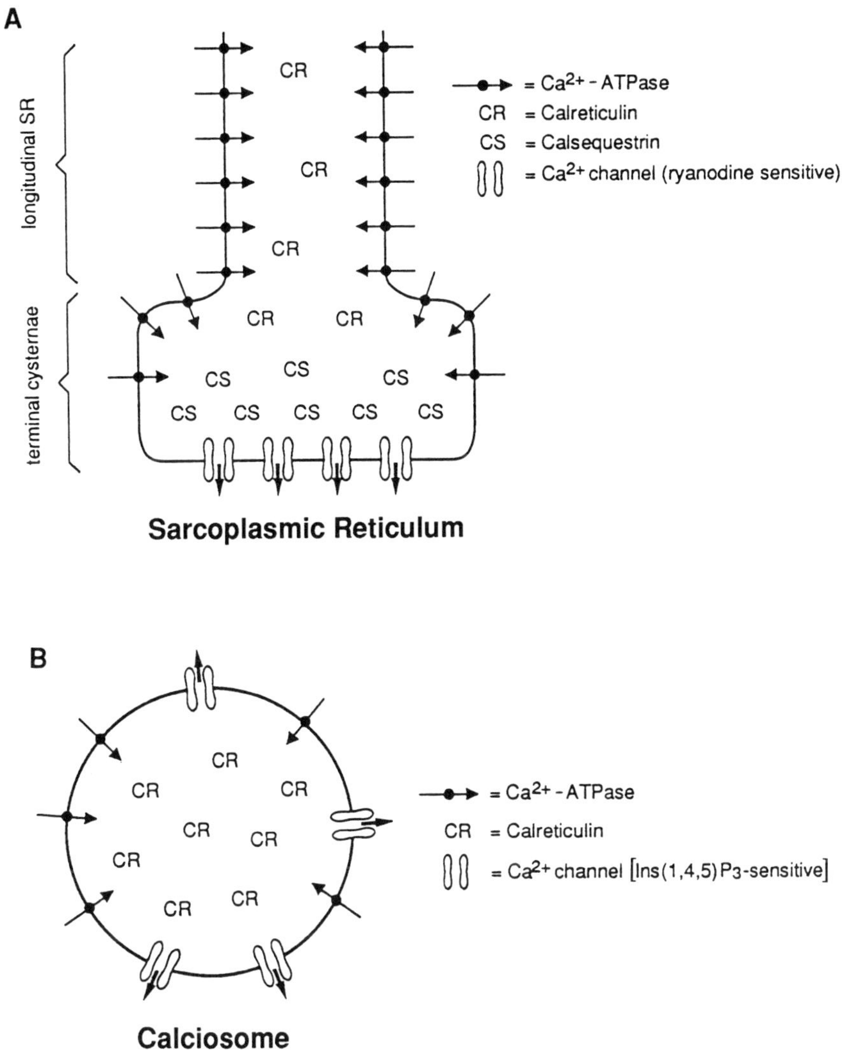

FIGURE 2

Intracellular Ca^{2+} stores of muscle [i.e., sarcoplasmic reticulum (SR)] and HL-60 cells (i.e., calciosomes). (A) Muscle SR consists of two compartments that are continuous *in vivo,* but separately recovered in subcellular fractionation studies: longitudinal SR (light SR) and terminal cysternae (heavy SR). The ryanodine-sensitive Ca^{2+} channel and calsequestrin are concentrated in the terminal cysternae, while the Ca^{2+}-ATPase and calreticulin are found in both compartments. (B) Subcellular fractionation studies in HL-60 cells have so far yielded a homogeneous recovery of markers of Ins(1,4,5)P_3-sensitive Ca^{2+} stores (i.e., calciosomes). Although calciosomes are recovered after separation of homogenates as small light-density vesicles (as shown), their relationship to other organelles (e.g., endoplasmic reticulum) has not yet been clarified.

(2) Ca^{2+} uptake can be inhibited by millimolar, not micromolar, concentrations of vanadate; and (3) Ca^{2+} uptake is not inhibited by calmodulin inhibitors. Immunological studies in HL-60 cells show an approximately 100-kDa protein that cross-reacts with monoclonal antibodies against slow-twitch/cardiac Ca^{2+}-ATPase, but not fast-twitch Ca^{2+}-ATPase (18). The subcellular distribution of this protein parallels the distribution of Ca^{2+} pumping and Ins(1,4,5)P_3 response in subcellular fractions of HL-60 cells (18). It is thus likely that this protein is the Ca^{2+} pump of the intracellular Ca^{2+} store in HL-60 cells. This assumption is supported by studies in liver and pancreas showing a phosphorylated intermediate of a Ca^{2+}-ATPase with a molecular mass similar to that of the HL-60 protein (93, 94). However, purification of the enzyme and functional studies is necessary to define more precisely the role of this protein in HL-60 cells.

Ca^{2+} Release Channels (InsP_3-Sensitive, Ryanodine Sensitive, Caffeine Sensitive)

An Ins(1,4,5)P_3-sensitive Ca^{2+} channel has been purified and cloned from mouse cerebellum (95). This channel has some homology with the ryanodine-sensitive Ca^{2+} channel of muscle cells. Thus, there seems to be a genetically related family of intracellular Ca^{2+} release channels. Primary structures of Ca^{2+} release channels from tissues other than muscle or nerve have not been reported so far; however, mRNA of an appropriate size that cross-hybridizes with cDNA of the cerebellar InsP_3 receptor has been found in a variety of tissues (96).

Recent patch–clamp studies show the existence of a voltage-dependent caffeine-sensitive Ca^{2+} release channel in ER preparations of pancreatic cells (97). This channel seems to be insensitive to Ins(1,4,5)P_3 and the cytosolic free Ca^{2+}. It might be a Ca^{2+} release channel of an Ins(1,4,5)P_3-insensitive Ca^{2+} store. No information is presently available on the biochemical properties of the intracellular Ca^{2+} release channel of human neutrophils.

Intravesicular Ca^{2+} Storage Proteins

The sarcoplasmic reticulum of skeletal and cardiac muscle contains at least two proteins that bind Ca^{2+} with high capacity but low affinity and might therefore function as intravesicular Ca^{2+} storage proteins: calsequestrin and calreticulin (Fig. 2). Calreticulin is also found in a variety of nonmuscle cells, while calsequestrin seems to be exclusively expressed in nonmuscle cells (98). As discussed above, the Ins(1,4,5)P_3-responsive subcellular fractions in HL-60 cells are enriched in a 60-kDa Ca^{2+}-binding protein. We have purified this protein and shown that its N-terminal amino acid sequence has 93% similarity to calreticulin (99).

Thus, calreticulin is likely to function as a Ca^{2+} storage protein of the Ins(1,4,5)P_3-sensitive Ca^{2+} stores of HL-60 cells. No Ca^{2+}-binding data of the HL-60 protein are available so far. However, the muscle calreticulin has been shown to possess approximately 20 low-affinity binding sites and one or two high-affinity binding sites. While the physiological role of the low-affinity binding sites is likely to be Ca^{2+} storage, nothing is known about the potential physiological role of the high-affinity binding site.

Muscle calreticulin has the C-terminal amino acid sequence KDEL (in single-letter code), which is referred to as the "retention sequence for luminal ER proteins" (98). While most luminal proteins that do not possess this sequence are transported from the ER via the cis-Golgi and trans-Golgi to their final destination, proteins with the KDEL sequence are either directly retained within the ER or retransported from the cis-Golgi to the ER (100) (Fig. 3). As calreticulin has a Golgi-typical glycosylation pattern (101), it is most likely transported through the latter pathway.

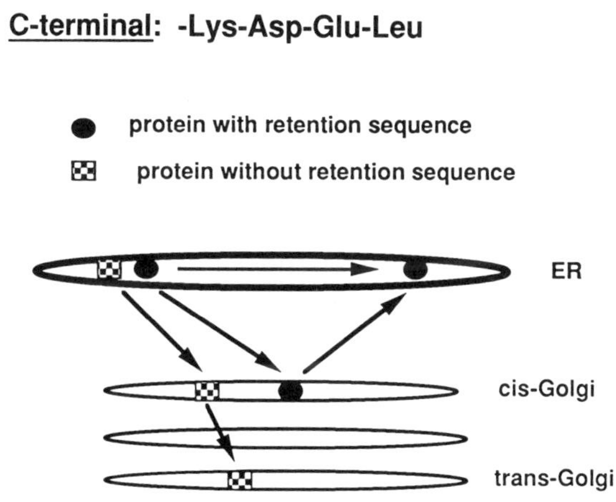

FIGURE 3

Endoplasmic reticulum (ER) retention sequence. Recent studies on the sorting of luminal proteins in the ER (for a review see Ref. 100) have suggested a C-terminal sequence of Lys–Asp–Glu–Leu (KDEL in single-letter code). Most luminal proteins without this retention sequence pass through the cis-Golgi via trans-Golgi to their final destination. Proteins with the C-terminal KDEL sequence are either directly retained within the ER or pass through the cis-Golgi and are subsequently retransported to the ER.

Model of Biosynthesis of Calciosomes and Their Relationship to the ER

Although the C-terminal sequence of the calreticulin-related protein of HL-60 cells is not yet known, so far there is no evidence that it differs from that of muscle calreticulin. Thus, on the one hand calreticulin is presumably retained in the ER via a KDEL sequence (see the previous section). On the other hand, however, it is not recovered together with typical ER markers (e.g., NADPH–cytochrome *c* reductase and sulfatase C) in subcellular fractionation studies. This apparent contradiction might be explained by the following model of calciosome biosynthesis (Fig. 4).

Calciosome proteins are synthesized in the ER, with a possible passage through the Golgi apparatus. In a second step they are concentrated within

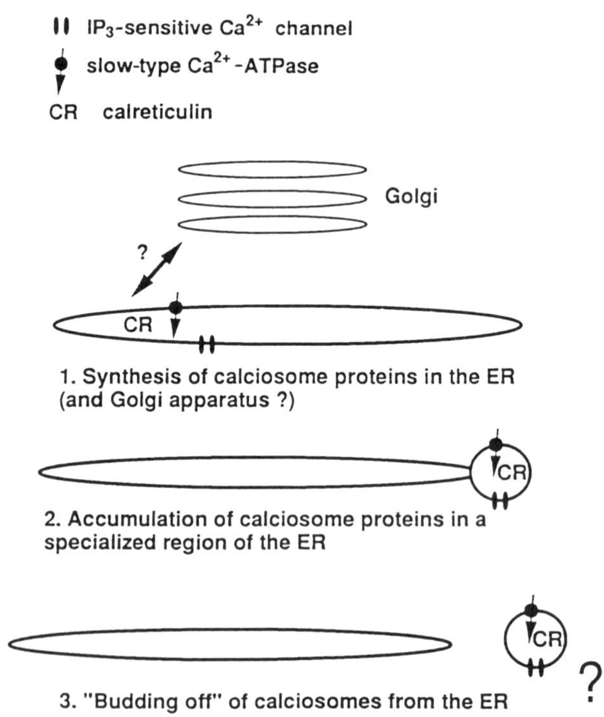

FIGURE 4

Possible model of the biosynthesis of calciosomes. Calciosome proteins are synthesized in the endoplasmic reticulum (ER) (1) and after a passage through the cis-Golgi are concentrated in a specialized region of the ER. Calciosomes might be *in vivo* continuous (2) or discontinuous (3) with the ER.

a portion of the ER, and finally a "budding off" of calciosomes from the ER occurs. The second step must occur in order to explain the results of the above described subcellular fractionation studies in HL-60 cells; that is, the bulk of the ER does not copurify with markers of intracellular Ca^{2+} stores. However, so far there is no proof that the third step (i.e., the budding off) occurs *in vivo*. Calciosomes and ER might be distinct but continuous structures in intact HL-60 cells, and their physical separation might be due to the homogenization procedure. This would resemble the situation in muscle cells, in which the terminal cysternae and the longitudinal SR are recovered in different subcellular fractions, but are thought to be continuous structures *in vivo*.

Thus, while the existence of a specialized Ins(1,4,5)P_3-responsive structure in HL-60 cells (i.e., the calciosome) is clearly demonstrated by the results of the subcellular fractionation studies, the *in vivo* relationship to other organelles, particularly the ER, needs further investigation. Morphological electron microscopic studies attempting three-dimensional reconstruction of calciosomes will be particularly important.

Phosphatidylinositol Turnover

The formation and metabolism of inositol polyphosphates are complex processes that occur in a wide variety of cells (27) (Fig. 5). Two types of kinases phosphorylate phosphatidylinositol (PtdIns) to yield several isomeric forms of the polyphosphatidylinositol lipids (e.g., PtdInsP, PtdInsP_2, and PtdInsP_3). The type I kinase produces PtdIns(3)P, PtdIns(3,4)P_2, and PtdIns(3,4,5)P_3. Interestingly, PtdIns(3,4)P_2, seems to be generated during the activation of neutrophils (29). However, the type I kinase products appear only after cell stimulation with growth factor-like substances in parallel with the activation of protein tyrosine kinases (102). In addition PtdIns(3)P, PtdIns(3,4)P_2, and PtdIns(3,4,5)P_3 are only poor substrates for at least four distinct isoenzymes of phospholipase C (103). The cleavage of the membrane phospholipid PtdIns(4,5)P_2 through the activation of the type II kinase is a widely distributed process. It constitutes a cornerstone of signaling mechanisms coupling a wide variety of stimuli to the activation of cells of different types, leading to the generation of the Ca^{2+}-mobilizing second messenger Ins(1,4,5)P_3 (9, 28, 104).

Ins(1,4,5)P_3 is further metabolized by a series of specific phosphomonoesterases and kinases (Fig. 5). The two key enzymes in this metabolism are Ins(1,4,5)P_3 5-phosphatase and Ins(1,4,5)P_3 3-kinase (7). The Ins(1,4,5)P_3 5 -phosphatase is likely to play an important role in termination of the

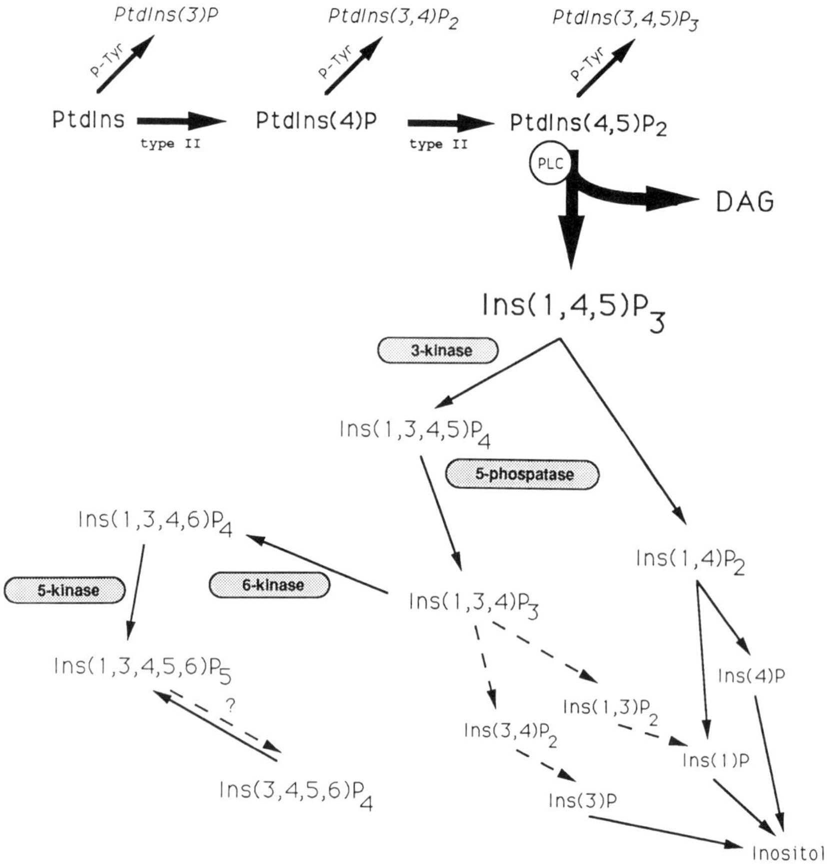

FIGURE 5

Cycle of phosphoinositides and inositol phosphates. This cycle involves (a) generation of phosphatidylinositol from inositol and diacylglycerol (DAG) in the endoplasmic reticuium, (b) generation of a variety of higher phosphorylated phosphoinositides by specific kinases, (c) generation of the cyclic alcohol Ins(1,4,5)P_3 by cleavage of phosphatidylinositol (4,5)-bisphosphate, and (d) further inositol phosphate metabolism by a series of specific kinases and phosphatases. PLC, Phospholipase C.

Ins(1,4,5)P_3 response by generating the inactive Ins(1,4)P_2 (105–107). Ins(1,4)P_2 degradation proceeds by sequential dephosphorylation through the activation of polyphosphomonoesterases and allows the subsequent regeneration and recycling of *myo*-inositol. The Ins(1,4,5)P_3 3-kinase specifically converts Ins(1,4,5)P_3 into Ins(1,3,4,5)P_4 (108). The affinity of this enzyme for Ins(1,4,5)P_3 is almost 10-fold higher than that of the

Ins(1,4,5)P_3 5-phosphatase. The affinity for Ins(1,4,5)P_3 of the partially purified enzyme in HL-60 cells was 0.4 μM (D. Pittet and D. P. Lew, unpublished observations), consistent with values obtained in other cellular systems. Its activity is regulated by the Ca^{2+} calmodulin complex (109, 110) and possibly also by phosphorylation (111). Following cell surface receptor occupancy the activity of the Ins(1,4,5)P_3 3-kinase and 5-phosphatase drives the metabolism to the tris/tetrakisphosphate pathway. The subsequent metabolism of Ins(1,4,5)P_3 and Ins(1,3,4,5)P_4 seems thus to be intricate. The reasons for the complex metabolic pathway leading to the generation of multiple inositol phosphates are still unclear. Experimental evidence suggests a function in the regulation of $[Ca^{2+}]_i$ for certain isomers (e.g., Ins(1,3,4,5)P_4), but the contributions of inositol phosphates other than Ins(1,4,5)P_3 remain to be defined. However, the extra energy expenditure required to produce Ins(1,3,4,5)P_4, as well as other highly phosphorylated InsPs, supports their involvement in regulation of as yet undefined cellular functions.

The actual view of the inositol phosphate metabolism suggested the existence of two functional groups of inositol phosphates: agonist sensitive and agonist insensitive (27). The inositol phosphates of the first group are supposed to have functions related to cell signaling. The proposed roles for Ins(1,3,4,5)P_4 include modulation of $[Ca^{2+}]_i$ through the reuptake of Ca^{2+} into intracellular stores, control of the Ca^{2+} transfer process between Ins(1,4,5)P_3-sensitive and -insensitive pools, the modulation of Ca^{2+} influx across the plasma membrane, or the potentiation of Ins(1,4,5)P_3-induced Ca^{2+} mobilization. Different aspects of the metabolism of Ins(1,3,4,5)P_4 in HL-60 cells strongly supports its potential role as an intracellular messenger. Detailed analysis of Ins(1,3,4,5)P_4 generation revealed (1) rapid kinetics following agonist stimulation: (2) a dose-dependent relationship, with very high sensitivity to low agonist concentrations; and (3) $[Ca^{2+}]_i$-dependent accumulation (75). These observations were made by using an optimized high-performance liquid chromatography procedure for the separation of the three distinct inositol tetrakisphosphate isomers [Ins(1,3,4,6)P_4, Ins(1,3,4,5)P_4, and Ins(3,4,5,6)P_4]. Marked differences were noted in the kinetics, dose dependence, and $[Ca^{2+}]_i$ sensitivity of these isomers following cell surface receptor activation. Moreover, when absolute intracellular concentrations of Ins(1,4,5)P_3 and Ins(1,3,4,5)P_4 were quantified in HL-60 cells [using the metal dye detection technique (see below)], the levels of the latter rose faster than those of any other inositol phosphate. In addition, the increase in the intracellular concentration of Ins(1,3,4,5)P_4 was similar in magnitude to the changes occurring in its precursor, Ins(1,4,5)P_3, or for the product arising from its dephosphorylation, Ins(1,3,4)P_3. This supports the presumption that, following receptor activation, Ins(1,4,5)P_3 is metabolized via phosphorylation rather than dephosphorylation.

Ins(1,3,4,5)P_4 is only one of several highly phosphorylated inositol phosphates that may increase upon receptor stimulation. At least Ins(1,3,4,6)P_4 and Ins(1,3,4,5,6)P_5 result from Ins(1,3,4,5)P_4 metabolism, highlighting the importance of the initial drive through the $InsP_3/P_4$ pathway (112). However, studies of inositol phosphate metabolism are generally performed using steady-state radioactive labeling of the inositol phospholipids and inositol phosphates, presumably approaching isotopic equilibrium. Using a newly developed procedure, the metal dye detection technique, we could quantify absolute concentrations of InsPs in HL-60 cells (113). This analysis revealed unexpected changes in highly phosphorylated InsPs. Absolute intracellular concentration of Ins(1,3,4,5,6)P_5, an isomer which, in the past, was assumed to be unaffected by agonist stimulation (when assessed using radiotracer methods), showed marked increased upon fMLP stimulation in HL-60 cells. Importantly, Ins(1,3,4,5,6)P_5 levels were 36 μM in resting cells [100-fold higher than the levels of Ins(1,4,5)P_3] and increased to more than 50 μM 1 min after agonist stimulation. These variations represent a more significant mass change in absolute terms for Ins(1,3,4,5,6)P_5 than for any other InsP. The physiological significance of these observations remains to be studied.

Recent studies have suggested the existence of metabolically distinct pools of precursor phospholipids. Thus, methods that quantify the real concentration of both inositol phospholipids and inositol phosphates, rather than incorporation of radioactivity, become increasingly important. Using metal dye detection analysis, we recently identified "new" inositol phosphates that had not been described in radiotracer studies (114). Moreover, mass analysis using radiolabeled cells revealed differences in the specific radioactivity of various groups of inositol phosphates and marked changes upon agonist stimulation in a subset of inositol phosphates (113). These observations strongly support the existence of different pools of inositol phosphates with multiple pathways stimulated during cell activation. Moreover, it appears that inositol phosphates should certainly not only be defined as a function of their agonist sensitivity, but also as members of "families" whose size and role must be studied.

Thus, inositol phosphates might form a family of intracellular messengers which regulate $[Ca^{2+}]_i$ and possibly other cellular processes (e.g., $InsP_5$ and $InsP_6$ modulate the oxygen affinity of hemoglobin in birds). Differences in $InsP_5$ and $InsP_6$ levels at different stages of differentiation have been demonstrated in oocytes (112). In HL-60 cells the levels of the highly phosphorylated InsPs change during cell differentiation, suggesting a role in trophic regulation and/or cell adaptation (R. H. Michell, personal communication). Interestingly, highly phosphorylated inositol phosphates have been shown to bind aldolases with high affinity, leading to an inhibition of the enzyme activity (115). Some InsPs might thus represent allosteric regulators of intracellular enzymes. The role of highly phosphorylated InsPs in gene regulation deserves further investigation; for example, Ins(1,4,5)P_3 3-kinase activity is increased in v-*src*-transformed cells (116). Finally, it has been suggested that $InsP_5$ and $InsP_6$ are extracellular signals (117). In human neutrophils we were not able to demonstrate either inositol phosphate secretion by chemoattractant-stimulated cells or any concentration gradient in subcellular fractions (D. Pittet, unpublished observations).

Role of $[Ca^{2+}]_i$ in the Regulation of Neutrophil Functions

Regulation of Exocytosis by $[Ca^{2+}]_i$

The term "exocytosis" is commonly used to indicate the process by which hydrophilic cellular products (e.g., proteins, peptides, and neurotransmitters) segregated within intracellular vesicles are discharged into the extracellular fluid. This process is triggered by stimulation of the cell and consists of several discrete events, including the movement of the storage organelles to the plasma membrane, fusion between the two membranes, and liberation of the stored contents. In phagocytes a particular form of exocytosis exists in which the content of granules is discharged into the phagosome. Thus, although the granule content is discharged within the cells, phagosome–lysosome fusion bears many similarities to the exocytotic process in other cellular systems.

More than 20 years ago it was discovered that Ca^{2+} plays a pivotal role in regulated exocytosis. In particular it has been demonstrated that exocytosis often depends on the presence of Ca^{2+} in the extracellular medium and that it can be induced by ionophores that selectively transport Ca^{2+} across natural and artificial membranes (118, 119). Additional support for the involvement of Ca^{2+} has been provided by the discovery of the inhibitory action of Ca^{2+} antagonists and the role of Ca^{2+}-regulated proteins (119–121). In recent years two technical developments have led to important progress in this field, namely, the introduction of permeabilized cells that retain their capacity to secrete (122–124) and the use of fluorescent Ca^{2+} chelators for manipulating and measuring cytosolic free calcium concentration $[Ca^{2+}]_i$ (43, 125). The quantitative relationship between $[Ca^{2+}]_i$

and secretion has been investigated in permeabilized cells, and, more recently, validation of such data has been performed in our laboratory on intact cells (44, 125, 126).

In this section we summarize results obtained by two different methodologies for the investigation of the $[Ca^{2+}]_i$ dependency of exocytosis in intact human neutrophils: (1) introduction of high-affinity Ca^{2+} chelators (e.g., quin2 and MAPT) into intact cells to buffer and control $[Ca^{2+}]_i$ transients and (2) establishment of $[Ca^{2+}]_i$ steady state with the Ca^{2+} ionophore ionomycin. Before summarizing these results a word of caution should be applied: An important part of the methodology described here has been used in populations of human neutrophils in suspension. We have more recently discovered that surface-adherent neutrophils behave differently in their properties, particularly regarding their Ca^{2+} homeostasis when compared to the same cells in suspension.

Studies in Neutrophils in Suspension

The introduction of a new generation of Ca^{2+} indicators of high affinity and selectivity, the tetracarboxylates, and their intercellularly hydrolyzable alkyl esters allowed the determination of $[Ca^{2+}]_i$ in small intact mammalian cells. Initially, quin2 was the most useful of the tetracarboxylate Ca^{2+} indicators; in most cases it has been used either nonquantitatively or simply to demonstrate $[Ca^{2+}]_i$ rises as a consequence of certain stimuli (125, 127–129). Afterward quin2 was used as a high-affinity Ca^{2+} chelator to buffer and control $[Ca^{2+}]_i$ transients, while simultaneously monitoring the actual values of $[Ca^{2+}]_i$ (130–132). Some of the more representative experiments performed in populations of human neutrophils are described below.

Three subcellular compartments have been shown to release their content into the extracellular medium and were therefore studied. They are, respectively (a convenient marker is indicated in parentheses), primary granules (β-glucuronidase), secondary granules (vitamin B_{12}-binding protein), and secretory vesicles (gelatinase).

Effect of intracellular $[quin2]_i$ on $[Ca^{2+}]_i$ Transients Induced by the Chemotactic Peptide fMLP. In Ca^{2+} medium at low $[quin2]_i$ there is a rapid increase in $[Ca^{2+}]_i$ that reaches micromolar levels, followed by a progressive decrease to basal levels. At high $[quin1]_i$ the amplitude of the $[Ca^{2+}]_i$ rise is markedly reduced, usually reaching values no higher than 2- or 3-fold the basal values (e.g., at its maximum, ~300 n*M*). The kinetics of the $[Ca^{2+}]_i$ transients are very different at high or low quin2 loadings. At low loading, upon addition of fMLP, there is a rapid rise that is completed in less than 10 sec, followed by a slow return to the basal level. At high loading the rapid phase is drastically reduced in amplitude, and a slow phase of $[Ca^{2+}]_i$ rise is then observed that lasts for over 4 min. The fast component must be attributed to the release of Ca^{2+} from intracellular stores, since it is also observed in the presence of EGTA, while the slow component is probably due to an increased influx from the extracellular medium, since it is abolished when external Ca^{2+} is removed.

While at low $[quin2]_i$ loadings in Ca^{2+}-free medium, an important $[Ca^{2+}]_i$ rise can still be measured (up to 850 n*M*); at high loadings the $[Ca^{2+}]_i$ rise is barely significant, from 90 to 115 n*M*. The differences in $[Ca^{2+}]_i$ rise at high and low loading in Ca^{2+}-free medium should be attributed to the different Ca^{2+}-buffering capacity provided by quin2, since the amount of Ca^{2+} released in the two cases is rather similar.

We tested in parallel, in the same batch of cells, the effect of $[quin2]_i$ on granule content release induced by fMLP. Increasing $[quin2]_i$ decreases the amount of primary and secondary granule exocytoses in Ca^{2+} medium. The inhibitory effect on granule content release is much more pronounced in Ca^{2+}-free medium, even in cells loaded with the lowest $[quin2]_i$.

Effect of $[quin2]_i$ on $[Ca^{2+}]_i$ Transients Induced by the Calcium Ionophore Ionomycin. quin2 affects $[Ca^{2+}]_i$ rise induced by the calcium ionophore ionomycin in a predictable way: In Ca^{2+} medium increasing quin2 loadings decreases the rate of $[Ca^{2+}]_i$ rise without affecting its final extent. In contrast, the rate of $[Ca^{2+}]_i$ increase in Ca^{2+}-free medium is practically unaffected by the extent of $[quin2]_i$, while the magnitude of the $[Ca^{2+}]_i$ rise is dramatically decreased. Again, the difference must be ascribed to the extra cytosolic Ca^{2+}-buffering capacity provided by quin2, since the amount of Ca^{2+} released is similar at both high and low loadings.

Effect of $[quin2]_i$ on $[Ca^{2+}]_i$ in the Absence of Extracellular Ca^{2+}. Levels of $[Ca^{2+}]_i$ below the resting level were obtained by loading the cells with quin2 in Ca^{2+}-free medium (133). Under these conditions the Ca^{2+} stores are depleted, and basal $[Ca^{2+}]_i$ is decreased 3- to 10-fold below the normal resting level, depending on the $[quin2]_i$ used. This last approach has proved extremely useful for determining whether a process under study is Ca^{2+} dependent or independent, since, at resting $[Ca^{2+}]_i$ levels below 20 n*M*, Ca^{t+}-dependent processes do not occur.

Establishment of $[Ca^{2+}]_i$ Steady State with the Calcium Ionophore Ionomycin in Ca^{2+}-Buffered Cells. A second experimental approach which proved most useful was to establish $[Ca^{2+}]_i$ steady state in neutrophils with a calcium ionophore and to assess the effect of different $[Ca^{2+}]_i$ values obtained on secretion.

The cells were loaded with the Ca^{2+} chelator and indicator quin2, $[Ca^{2+}]_i$ steady states were established with a fixed concentration of ionomycin (500 n*M*) and different concentrations of extracellular Ca^{2+}, and exocytosis from three distinct subcellular storage organelles was assessed.

Ionomycin induced a rapid rise in $[Ca^{2+}]_i$ up to a plateau which depended on the $[Ca^{2+}]_i$. The plateau remained constant for 10 min, indicating that steady-state levels ranging from 120 to over 2000 n*M* can be established by the experimental protocol adopted. Due to the poor indicator sensitivity of quin2 at $[Ca^{2+}]_i$ above 2 μ*M*, calibration at higher values should not be attempted.

Conclusions about the Usefulness of This Approach for the Study of $[Ca^{2+}]_i$ in Exocytosis of Neutrophils in Suspension. Human neutrophils are ideal as a model cell to study the $[Ca^{2+}]_i$ dependency of exocytosis, because they contain three biochemically well-defined storage compartments with different reactivity to exocytotic stimuli (134–136).

We have addressed the question of whether Ca^{2+} plays a role in neutrophil activation by using two different methodologies. The first was by trapping into the cytoplasm of neutrophils various concentrations of the Ca^{2+} indicator quin2, which binds Ca^{2+} with high affinity. This allowed us experimentally to increase progressively the cytosolic Ca^{2+}-buffering capacity and subsequently to monitor the kinetics of $[Ca^{2+}]_i$ rises and functional response induced by fMLP or ionomycin.

In the case of exocytosis there was a clear-cut correlation between the final extent of $[Ca^{2+}]_i$ rise and exocytosis of the contents of both primary (β-glucuronidase) and secondary (vitamin B_{12}-binding protein) granules. Increasing $[quin2]_i$ decreases the maximal $[Ca^{2+}]_i$ rises and exocytosis in response to fMLP, and these decreases are even more pronounced in Ca^{2+}-free buffer, in which Ca^{2+} influx from the extracellular medium is negligible and Ca^{2+} originates only from intracellular pools. The calcium ionophore ionomycin, which bypasses membrane surface receptors and tends to dissipate $[Ca^{2+}]_i$ gradients (132), causes rapid rises in $[Ca^{2+}]_i$ and degranulation at low quin2 loadings. Increasing quin2 loadings progressively decreases the rates of $[Ca^{2+}]_i$ rises and exocytosis induced by the ionophore, but since, in contrast to fMLP, the effects of the ionophore are sustained, eventually both parameters tend to reach maximal levels. This approach allowed the demonstration that there is a Ca^{2+} dependency for exocytosis in human neutrophils.

The second methodology was to use a calcium ionophore to obtain different $[Ca^{2+}]_i$ steady states and thus quantify more properly the Ca^{2+} dependency of secretion.

Minimal enzyme release was observed when $[Ca^{2+}]_i$ was less than 200–

250 n*M*. Above this level release occurred, albeit to different extents, from all three storage compartments. From the same experiments the $[Ca^{2+}]_i$ that gave half-maximal release (EC_{50}) of three markers was calculated. In neutrophils pretreated with cytochalasin B, these values were 610 and 650 n*M* for vitamin B_{12}-binding protein and gelatinase, respectively (no statistical difference). The EC_{50} for β-glucuronidase release was 2600 n*M*, which is much higher than the EC_{50} for release from specific granules and secretory vesicles. $[Ca^{2+}]_i$ threshold and EC_{50} for exocytosis from specific granules and secretory vesicles were similar.

The "ionophore clamp" approach overcomes some of the problems found in the studies with permeabilized cells, since it manipulates $[Ca^{2+}]_i$ more selectively. However, several factors (i.e., Ca^{2+} release from intracellular stores, Ca^{2+} buffering, and the effect of pH gradients across the membrane) must be taken into consideration, and reliable information can be obtained only if $[Ca^{2+}]_i$ is monitored. It must be noted that ionophore clamping assumes that the ionophore can completely overcome the Ca^{2+}-buffering mechanisms of the cell, so that $[Ca^{2+}]_i$ = 2-Δ-pH $[Ca^{2+}]_i$. We observed that with 0.5–1.0 μ*M* ionomycin $[Ca^{2+}]_o$ was still ~1000-fold higher than $[Ca^{2+}]_i$, and the equilibrium $[Ca^{2+}]_i$ = 2-Δ-pH $[Ca^{2+}]_i$ was not reached, even at 10 μ*M* ionomycin. The approach used in this study is related to the ionophore clamp method. The high-affinity Ca^{2+} chelator quin2 served two purposes: it allowed manipulation of $[Ca^{2+}]_i$ and monitoring of these levels. Another useful alternative approach is to combine the fluorescent Ca^{2+}-sensitive probe fura-2 with an intracellular nonfluorescent Ca^{2+} chelator such as MAPT. In summary this approach offers several advantages, particularly for the study of single cells. This approach allowed us not only to find that chemoattractant-triggered secretion is a Ca^{2+}-dependent process, but also to quantify the $[Ca^{2+}]_i$ requirement for half-maximal exocytosis. The EC_{50}s of specific granules and secretory vesicles were significantly lower than that for azurophil granules (Fig. 6).

Studies in Adherent Neutrophils

Buffering $[Ca^{2+}]_i$ Transients and Assessment of Exocytosis at the Single-Cell Level in Adherent Neutrophils. The approach described in the previous section was naturally attempted in adherent neutrophils. However, we realized that several properties of the $[Ca^{2+}]_i$ signal were different in adherent neutrophils. First was the unexpected discovery of the presence of spontaneous $[Ca^{2+}]_i$ oscillations not observed previously in cells in suspension. Second, the addition of EGTA to the extracellular medium led

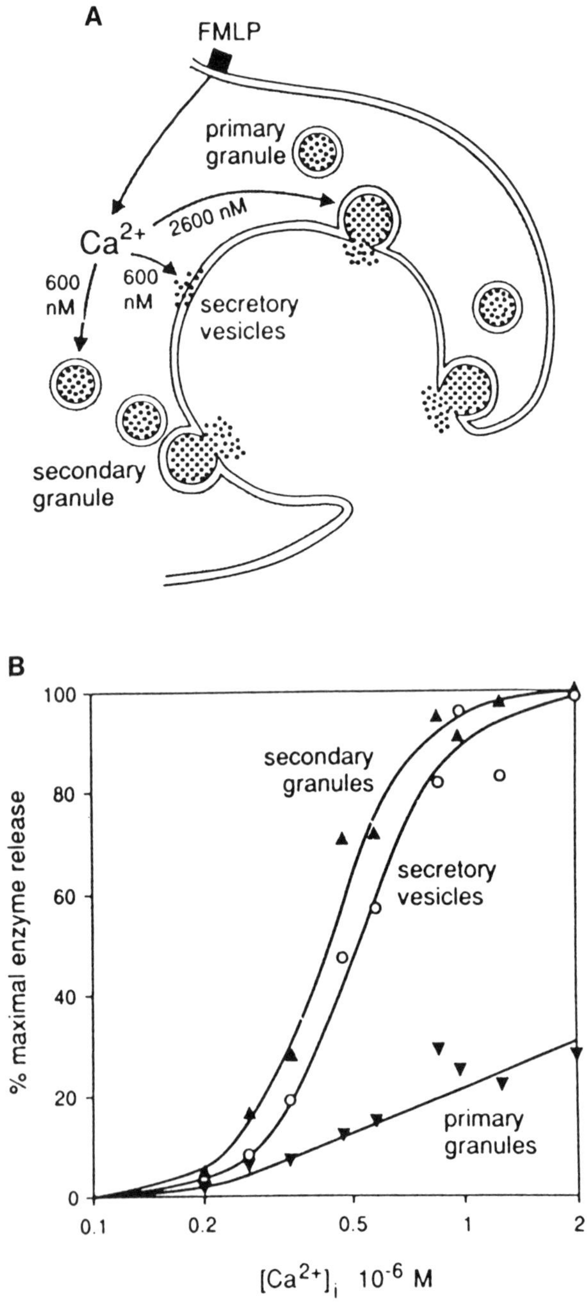
A
FMLP
primary
granule
Ca^{2+}
2600 nM
600
nM
600
nM
secretory
vesicles
secondary
granule
B
100
80
60
40
20
0
% maximal enzyme release
secondary
granules
secretory
vesicles
primary
granules
0.1
0.2
0.5
1
2
$[Ca^{2+}]_i$ 10^{-6} M

to rapid intracellular Ca^{2+} store depletion, a marked difference when compared to cells in suspension in which Ca^{2+} stores remain full for several hours in the presence of Ca^{2+} chelators in the extracellular medium. Taking these differences into account, a similar methodology for $[Ca^{2+}]_i$ manipulation could be achieved.

We have monitored in parallel at the single-cell level $[Ca^{2+}]_i$ transients during phagocytosis and accumulation of lactoferrin within the phagocytic vesicle (i.e., the fusion of secondary granules with the phagocytic vesicle) by immunofluorescent staining. These experiments were performed under three conditions: (1) normal control cells in the presence of extracellular Ca^{2+}, (2) cells with increased cytosolic buffering capacity, and (3) $[Ca^{2+}]_i$-depleted cells (MAPT loading in the presence or absence of Ca^{2+}, respectively). Discharge of granule content into the phagosome was detected in 80% of the control cells as a highly fluorescent ring around the ingested particle. This percentage was reduced to 30% in Ca^{2+}-buffered cells and further to less than 10% in Ca^{2+}-depleted cells (48).

We could thus show at the single-cell level that $[Ca^{2+}]_i$ elevations are not necessary for ingestion of particles, but control the fusion of granules with the phagocytic vesicle during phagocytosis in human neutrophils (48). These experiments indicate that the approach described above for large populations of cells can also be used at the single-cell level (and even at a subcellular level with image analysis systems in the future) for assessment of the role of Ca^{2+} in the control of secretion. It has been suggested in other cellular systems that the control of secretion is frequency encoded; that is, it is not only the amplitude, but also the frequency, of $[Ca^{2+}]_i$ spiking that determines the rate and extent of secretion. The precise role of these $[Ca^{2+}]_i$ transients in modulating secretion in neutrophils remains to be determined.

Role of Ca^{2+} in Chemotaxis and Phagocytosis

Clearly, $[Ca^{2+}]_i$ controls the "secretory code" of neutrophils. In contrast the role of $[Ca^{2+}]_i$ in modulating cell motile events has been more difficult to

FIGURE 6

Ca^{2+} dependency of exocytosis from three subcellular compartments in neutrophils. (A) Ca^{2+} regulates chemoattractant-triggered secretion with different Ca^{2+} dependencies for various granule populations. fMLP, f–Met–Leu–Phe. (B) Secretion of primary and secondary granules and secretory vesicle content at various steady-state $[Ca^{2+}]_i$ levels. [Reprinted with permission from D. P. Lew, *Eur. J. Clin. Invest.* **19**, 338–346 (1989).]

analyze. Phagocytosis of C3bi-coated yeasts in suspension is a Ca^{2+}-independent event, while $[Ca^{2+}]_i$ elevations are required to modulate this event if the yeast particle is coated with immunoglobulin G (137). When the neutrophils adhere, $[Ca^{2+}]_i$-independent ingestion, even of unopsonized particles, occurs (O. Stendahl *et al.*, unpublished observations). A similar complex relationship in $[Ca^{2+}]_i$ signaling occurs during chemotaxis.

Zigmond *et al.* (138) have shown that chemotaxis can occur in Ca^{2+}-depleted and/or -buffered cells. In contrast, Southwick *et al.* (139) have shown that, while spreading occurs in the absence of extracellular Ca^{2+}, adherence-associated actin polymerization on the lamellipodia requires the presence of this cation in the extracellular medium. Marks and Maxfield (140) suggested that $[Ca^{2+}]_i$ transients may play a role in the detachment of cells from protein-coated surfaces. Preliminary experiments from our laboratory suggest that, following attachment to a cell surface, upon subsequent spreading a series of $[Ca^{2+}]_i$ transients is generated. These $[Ca^{2+}]_i$ transients appear to result from activation of adherence receptors of the integrin family, particularly Mo1. Thus, the oscillatory component of $[Ca^{2+}]_i$ in neutrophils spreading or actively moving over surfaces appears to occur secondary to pseudopodal emission, contact with surfaces, and activation of adherence receptors. Ca^{2+} might not only help to control the actin network, but also regulate the localized secretion of granule components (resulting in proteolysis of extracellular matrix components) and deadhesion from the surface and killing of specific microbial targets.

Concluding Remarks

This review on Ca^{2+} translocation in signal transduction clearly witnesses the amazing complexity of the subject, even if the review had to be limited to only some aspects of this field. One might question whether this complexity of the Ca^{2+} signaling is really necessary for the appropriate regulation of neutrophil function. One might also argue, however, that what seems complicated to us is, in reality, the simplest solution of complicated problems. Taking the example of Ca^{2+} oscillation, the latter is likely to be the case. Until approximately 5 years ago almost any cell biologist would have predicted that the Ca^{2+} signal in nonexcitable cells is a process simply encoded by amplitude. The discovery of $[Ca^{2+}]_i$ oscillations in virtually all cell types has seriously questioned this assumption. Also, although the $[Ca^{2+}]_i$ oscillations were initially considered an "unnecessary complication," cell biologists learned through discussions with their colleagues in the engineering department what cells have probably known for millions of years: Frequency-encoded signals are more reliable and have less background noise than those encoded by amplitude. Thus, future research is likely to teach us how economical and straightforward the cellular strategies in Ca^{2+} signaling really are.

Acknowledgment

This work was supported by Swiss Research Foundation grant 32-30161.90.

References

1. B. M. Babior, *N. Engl. J. Med.* **298,** 721 (1978).
2. T. P. Stossel, *Semin. Hematol.* **12,** 83–116 (1975).
3. H. L. Malech and J. I. Gallin, *N. Engl. J. Med.* **317,** 687–694 (1987).
4. M. J. Berridge and R. F. Irvine, *Nature (London)* **312,** 315–320 (1984).
5. P. C. Downes and R. H. Michell, *in* "Molecular Mechanisms of Transmembrane Signalling" (P. Cohen and M. D. Houslay, eds.). Elsevier, Amsterdam, 1985.
6. B. Michell, *Nature (London)* **324,** 613 (1986).
7. T. M. Connolly, V. S. Bansal, T. E. Bross, R. F. Irvine, and P. W. Majerus, *J. Biol. Chem.* **262,** 2146–2149 (1987).
8. P. W. Majerus, T. M. Connolly, V. S. Bansal, R. C. Inhorn, and T. S. Ross, *J. Biol. Chem.* **263,** 3051–3054 (1988).
9. S. B. Shears, *Biochem. J.* **260,** 313–324 (1989).
10. S. B. Shears, *J. Biol. Chem.* **264,** 19879–19886 (1989).
11. A. E. Traynor-Kaplan, *Curr. Top. Membr. Transp.* **35,** 303–332 (1990).
12. R. Snyderman and R. J. Uhing, *in* "Inflammation: Basic Principles and Clinical Corraltes" (J. I. Gallin, I. M. Goldstein, and R. Snyderman, eds.), pp. 309–323. Raven, New York, 1988.
13. S. Cockcroft and B. D. Gomperts, *Nature (London)* **314,** 534–536 (1985).
14. M. M. Barrowman, S. Cockcroft, and B. D. Gomperts, *Nature (London)* **319,** 504–506 (1986).
15. L. A. Sklar, G. M. Bokoch, D. Button, and J. E. Smolen, *J. Biol. Chem.* **262,** 135–139 (1987).
16. G. M. Bokoch, *Curr. Top. Membr. Transp.* **35,** 65–101 (1990).
17. M. J. Berridge, P. H. Cobbold, and K. S. Cuthbertson, *Philos. Trans. R. Soc. London, Ser. B* **320,** 325–343 (1988).
18. K. H. Krause, D. Pittet, P. Volpe, J. Meldolesi, and D. P. Lew, *Cell Calcium* **10,** 351–361 (1989).
19. S. Shin, Y. Fujiwara, A. Wada, T. Takama, Y. Orita, T. Kamada, and K. Tagawa, *Biochem. Biophys. Res. Commun.* **142,** 70–77 (1987).
20. T. J. Rink, *FEBS Lett.* **268,** 381–385 (1990).
21. A. P. Morris, D. V. Gallacher, R. F. Irvine, and O. H. Petersen, *Nature (London)* **330,** 653–655 (1987).
22. R. F. Irvine, FEBS Lett. **263,** 5–9 (1990).

23. R. Y. Tsien, *Methods Cell Biol.* **30,** 127–156 (1989).
24. N. M. Woods, K. S. R. Cuthbertson, and P. H. Cobbold, *Cell Calcium* **8,** 79–100 (1987).
25. D. A. Williams, K. E. Fogarty, R. Y. Tsien, and F. S. Fay, *Nature (London)* **318,** 558–561 (1985).
26. J. H. Exton, *J. Biol. Chem.* **265,** 1–4 (1990).
27. M. J. Berridge and R. F. Irvine, *Nature (London* **341,** 197–205 (1989).
28. S. B. Dillon, J. J. Murray, R. J. Uhing, and R. Snyderman, *J. Cell. Biochem.* **35,** 345–359 (1987).
29. A. E. Traynor-Kaplan, B. L. Thompson, A. L. Harris, P. Taylor, G. M. Omann, and L. A. Sklar, *J. Biol. Chem.* **264,** 15668–15673 (1989).
30. L. Coussens, P. J. Parker, L. Rhee, T. L. Yang-Feng, E. Chen, M. D. Waterfield, U. Francke, and A. Ullrich, *Science* **233,** 859–866 (1986).
31. L. G. Rider and J. E. Niedel, *J. Biol. Chem.* **262,** 12015–12022 (1987).
32. A. Farago and Y. Nishizuka, *FEBS Lett.* **268,** 350–354 (1990).
33. M. Grzeskowiak, V. Della Bianca, M. A. Cassatella, and F. Rossi, *Biochem. Biophys. Res. Commun.* **135,** 785–794 (1986).
34. S. Grinstein and W. Furuya, *J. Biol. Chem.* **263,** 1779–1783 (1988).
35. H. M. Korchak, L. B. Vosshall, K. A. Haines, C. Wilkenfeld, K. F. Lundquist, and G. Weissmann, *J. Biol. Chem.* **263,** 11098–11105 (1988).
36. B. Dewald, M. Thelen, and M. Baggiolini, *J. Biol. Chem.* **263,** 16179–16184 (1988).
37. C. K. Huang, *Membr. Biochem.* **8,** 61–79 (1989).
38. P. E. Nasmith, G. B. Mills, and S. Grinstein, *Biochem. J.* **257,** 893–897 (1989).
39. W. L. Farrar, D. K. Ferris, D. F. Michiel, and D. Linnekin, *Curr. Top. Membr. Transp.* **35,** 425–467 (1990).
40. E. Sarndahl, M. Lindroth, T. Bengtsson, M. Fallmann, J. Gustavsson, O. Stendahl, and T. Andersson, *J. Cell Biol.* **109,** 279–284 (1989).
41. T. P. Stossel, *J. Biol. Chem.* **264,** 18261–18264 (1989).
42. T. P. Stossel, *in* "Inflammation: Basic Principles and Clinical Correlates" (J. I. Gallin, I. M. Goldstein, and R. Snyderman, eds.), pp. 325–342. Raven, New York, 1988.
43. T. Pozzan, P. D. Lew, C. B. Wollheim, and R. Y. Tsien, *Science* **221,** 1413–1415 (1983).
44. P. D. Lew, C. B. Wollheim, F. A. Waldvogel, and T. Pozzan, *J. Cell Biol.* **99,** 1212–1220 (1984).
45. P. D. Lew, *Eur. J. Clin. Invest.* **15,** 238–239 (1985).
46. B. A. Kruskal, S. Shak, and F. R. Maxfield, *Proc. Natl. Acad. Sci. U.S.A.* **83,** 2919–1923 (1986).
47. D. W. Sawyer, J. A. Sullivan, and G. L. Mandell, *Science* **230,** 663–666 (1985).
48. M. E. Jaconi, D. P. Lew, J. L. Carpentier, K. E. Magnusson, M. Sjögren, and O. Stendahl, *J. Cell Biol.* **110,** 1555–1564 (1990).
49. M. E. Jaconi, R. W. Rivest, W. Schlegel, C. B. Wollheim, D. Pittet, and P. D. Lew, *J. Biol. Chem.* **263,** 10557–10560 (1988).
50. T. Meyer and L. Stryer, *Proc. Natl. Acad. Sci. U.S.A.* **85,** 5051–5055 (1988).
51. M. Wakui, B. V. Potter, and O. H. Petersen, *Nature (London)* **339,** 317–320 (1989).
52. S. DeLisle, K.-H. Krause, G. Denning, B. V. L. Potter, and M. J. Welsh, *J. Biol. Chem.* **265,** 11726–11730 (1990).
53. L. Simchowitz and P. De Weer, *J. Gen. Physiol.* **88,** 167–181 (1986).
54. M. J. Welsh, *Physiol. Rev.* **67,** 1143–1162 (1987).
55. O. Christensen, *Nature (London)* **330,** 66–68 (1987).
56. D. T. Yamaguchi, J. Gree, C. R. Kleeman, and S. Muallem, *J. Biol. Chem.* **264,** 4383–4388 (1989).
57. H. M. Korchak and G. Weissman, *Proc. Natl. Acad. Sci. U.S.A.* **75,** 3818–3822 (1978).

58. M. Kuroki, N. Kamo, Y. Kobatake, E., Okimasu, and K. Utsumi, *Biochim. Biophys. Acta* **693,** 326 (1982).
59. B. E. Seligman, E. K. Gallin, D. L. Martin, W. Shain, and J. I. Gallin, *J. Membr. Biol.* **53,** 257 (1980).
60. C. L. Bashford and C. A. Pasternak, *Biochim. Biophys. Acta* **817,** 174–180 (1985).
61. M. A. Martin, W. M. Nauseef, and R. A. Clark, *J. Immunol.* **140,** 3928–3935 (1988).
62. L. M. Henderson, J. B. Chappell, and O. T. Jones, *Biochem. J.* **246,** 325–329 (1987).
63. K.-H. Krause and M. J. Welsh, *J. Clin. Invest.* **85,** 491–498 (1990).
64. N. S. Cook, *Trends Biochem. Sci.* **9,** 21–28 (1988).
65. T. Andersson, C. Dahlgren, T. Pozzan, O. Stendahl, and D. P. Lew, *Mol. Pharmacol.* **30,** 437–443 (1986).
66. F. Di Virgilio, P. D. Lew, T. Andersson, and T. Pozzan, *J. Biol. Chem.* **262,** 4574–4579 (1987).
67. D. Pittet, F. Di Virgilio, T. Pozzan, A. Monod, and D. P. Lew, *J. Biol. Chem.* (in press) (1990).
68. O. P. Hamill, A. Marty, E. Neher, B. Sakman, and F. Sigworth, *Pfluegers Arch.* **391,** 85 (1981).
69. E. Neher, *Neuroscience* **26,** 727–731 (1989).
70. M. Fletcher, *Arch. Microbiol.* **122,** 271–274 (1979).
71. E. K. Gallin, *Fed. Proc., Fed. Am. Soc. Exp. Biol.* **43,** 2385–2389 (1984) (abstr.).
72. V. von Tscharner, D. A. Deranleau, and M. Gaggiolini, *J. Biol. Chem.* **261,** 10163–10168 (1986).
73. V. von Tscharner, B. Prod'hom, M. Baggiolini, and H. Reuter, *Nature (London)* **324,** 369–372 (1986).
74. M. Kuno and P. Gardner, *Nature (London)* **326,** 301–304 (1987).
75. D. Pittet, D. P. Lew, G. W. Mayr, A. Monod, and W. Schlegel, *J. Biol. Chem.* **264,** 7251–7261 (1989).
76. P. M. Snyder, K.-H. Krause, and M. J. Welsh, *J. Biol. Chem.* **263,** 11048–11051 (1988).
77. H. Takemura, A. R. Hughes, O. Thastrup, and J. W. Putney, Jr., *J. Biol. Chem.* **264,**12266–12271 (1989).
78. C. Y. Kwan, H. Takemura, J. F. Obie, O. Thastrup, and J. W. Putney, Jr., *J. Cell. Physiol.* **27,** C1006–C1015 (1990).
79. H. Lagast, P. D. Lew, and F. A. Waldvogel, *J. Clin. Invest.* **73,** 107–115 (1984).
80. H. Lagast, T. Pozzan, F. A. Waldvogel, and P. D. Lew, *J. Clin. Invest.* **73,** 878–883 (1984).
81. A. K. Verma, A. G. Filoteo, D. R. Stanford, E. D. Wieben, J. Penniston, E. E. Strehler, R. Fischer, R. Heim, G. Vogel, S. Matthews, M.-A, Strehler-Page, P. James, T. Vorherr, J. Krebs, and E. Carafoli, *J. Biol. Chem.* **263,** 14152–14159 (1988).
82. R. O. Webster, I. M. Goldstein, and M. R. Flick, *J. Lab. Clin. Med.* **103,** 22–33 (1984).
83. P. Volpe, K.-H. Krause, S. Hashimoto, F. Zorzato, T. Pozzan, J. Meldolesi, and D. P. Lew, *Proc. Natl. Acad. Sci. U.S.A.* **85,** 1091–1095 (1988).
84. A. Amar-Costesec, M. Wibo, D. Thinès-Sempoux, H. Beaufay, and J. Berthet, *J. Cell Biol.* **62,** 717–745 (1974).
85. Y. Lange and T. L. Steck, *J. Biol. Chem.* **260,** 15592–15597 (1985).
86. I. Schulz, F. Thevenod, and M. Dehlinger Kremer, *Cell Calcium* **10,** 325–336 (1989).
87. T. R. Cheek, A. J. O'Sullivan, R. B. Moreton, M. J. Berridge, and R. D. Burgoyne, *FEBS Lett.* **266,** 91–95 (1990).
88. J. Lytton and D. H. MacLennan, *J. Biol. Chem.* **263,** 15024–15031 (1988).
89. A. M. Gunteski-Hamblin, J. Greeb, and G. E. Shull, *J. Biol. Chem.* **263,** 15032–15040 (1988).
90. R. D. Burgoyne, T. R. Cheek, A. Morgan, A. J. O'Sullivan, R. B. Moreton, M. J. Berridge, A. M. Mata, J. Coyler, A. G. Lee, and J. M. East, *Nature (London)* **343,** 72–74 (1989).

91. K.-H. Krause and P. D. Lew, *J. Clin. Invest.* **80,** 107–116 (1987).
92. M. Prentki, C. B. Wollheim, and P. D. Lew, *J. Biol. Chem.* **259,** 13777–13782 (1984).
93. C. Spanner, C. Heilmann, and W. Gerok, *J. Biol. Chem.* **262,** 7782–7789 (1987).
94. T. P. Kemmer, E. Bayerdorfer, H. Will, and I. Schulz, *J. Biol. Chem.* **262,** 13758–13764 (1987).
95. T. Furuichi, S. Yoshikawa, A. Miyawaki, K. Wasa, N. Maeda, and K. Mikoshiba, *Nature (London)* **342,** 32–38 (1989).
96. T. Furuichi, C. Shiota, and K. Mikoshiba, *FEBS Lett.* **267,** 85–88 (1990).
97. A. Schmidt, M. Dehlinger Kremer, I. Schulz, and H. Gögelein, *Nature (London)* **346,** 374 (1990).
98. L. Fliegel, K. Burns, D. H. MacLennan, R. A. F. Reithmeier, and M. Michalak, *J. Biol. Chem.* **264,** 21522–21528 (1989).
99. K.-H. Krause, K. B. Simmerman, L. R. Jones, and K. P. Campbell, *Biochem. J.* **270,** 545–548 (1990).
100. H. R. B. Pelham, *EMBO J.* **8,** 3171–3176 (1989).
101. P. Van Nguyen, F. Peter, and H.-D. Söling, *J. Biol. Chem.* **264,** 17494–17501 (1989).
102. K. R. Auger, L. A. Serunian, S. P. Soltoff, P. Libby, and L. C. Cantley, *Cell* **57,** 167–175 (1989).
103. L. A. Serunian, M. T. Haber, T. Fukui, J. Won Kim, S. Goo Rhee, J. M. Lowenstein, and J. C. Cantley, *J. Biol. Chem.* **264,** 17809–17815 (1989).
104. F. Di Virgilio, P. D. Lew, and T. Pozzan, *Biochem. Soc. Trans.* **12,** (1984).
105. T. M. Connolly, T. E. Bross, and P. W. Majerus, *J. Biol. Chem.* **260,** 7868–7874 (1985).
106. C. A. Hansen, R. A. Johanson, M. T. Williamson, and J. R. Williamson, *J. Biol. Chem.* **262,**17319–17326 (1987).
107. S. B. Shears, W. H. Evans, C. J. Kirk, and R. H. Michell, *Biochem. J.* **256,** 363–369 (1988).
108. R. F. Irvine, A. J. Letcher, J. P. Heslop, and M. J. Berridge, *Nature (London)* **320,** 631–634 (1986).
109. T. J. Biden, M. Comte, J. A. Cox, and C. B. Wollheim, *J. Biol. Chem.* **262,** 1–4 (1987).
110. T. J. Biden and C. B. Wollheim, *J. Biol. Chem.* **261,** 11931–11934 (1986).
111. K. Yamaguchi, M. Hirata, and H. Kuriyama, *Biochem. J.* **251,** 129–134 (1988).
112. H. Ji, K. Sandberg, A. J. Baukal, and K. J. Catt, *J. Biol. Chem.* **264,** 20185–20188 (1989).
113. D. Pittet, W. Schlegel, D. P. Lew, A. Monod, and G. W. Mayr, *J. Biol. Chem.* **264,** 18489–18493 (1989).
114. D. Pittet, G. W. Mayr, W. Schlegel, and P. D. Lew, manuscript in preparation (1991).
115. B. Koppitz, F. Vogel, and G. W. Mayr, *Eur. J. Biochem.* **161,** 421–433 (1986).
116. R. M. Johnson, W. J. Wasilenko, R. R. Mattingly, M. J. Weber, and J. C. Garrison, *Science* **246,** 121–124 (1989).
117. M. Vallejo, T. Jackson, S. Lightman, and M. R. Hanley, *Nature (London)* **330,** 656–658 (1987).
118. V. L. Lew and J. Garcia Sancho, *Methods* in "Enzymology" (S. Fleischer and B. Fleischer, eds.), Vol. 173, pp. 100–112. Academic Press, San Diego, California, 1989.
119. W. Y. Cheung, *Science* **207,** 19–25 (1980).
120. D. Romeo, G. Zabucchi, N. Miani, and F. Rossi, *Nature (London)* **253,** 542–544 (1975).
121. F. S. Southwick and T. P. Stossel, *Semin. Hematol.* **20,** 305–321 (1983).
122. P. F. Baker, D. E. Knight, and J. A. Umbach, *Cell Calcium* **6,** 5–14 (1985).
123. B. D. Gomperts, *Nature (London)* **306,** 64–66 (1983).
124. S. P. Nilson and N. Kishner, *J. Biol. Chem.* **258,** 4994–5000 (1983).
125. T. J. Rink, S. W. Smith, and R. Y. Tsien, *FEBS Lett.* **148,** 21–26 (1982).
126. P. D. Lew, A. Monod, F. A. Waldvogel, B. Dewald, M. Baggiolini, and T. Pozzan, *J. Cell Biol.* **102,** 2197–2204 (1986).

127. T. R. Hesketh, G. A. Smith, J. P. Moore, M. V. Taylor, and J. C. Metcalfe, *J. Biol. Chem.* **258,** 4876–4882 (1983).
128. J. R. White, P. H. Naccache, T. F. P. Molski, P. Borgeat, and R. I. Sha'afi, *Biochem. Biophys. Res. Commun.* **113,** 44–50 (1983).
129. C. B. Wollheim and T. Pozzan, *J. Biol. Chem.* **259,** 2262–2267 (1984).
130. V. L. Lew, R. Y. Tsien, C. Minex, and T. J. Rink, *Nature (London)* **298,** 478–481 (1982).
131. T. Pozzan, P. Arslan, R. Y. Tsien, and T. J. Rink, *J. Cell Biol.* **94,** 335–340 (1982).
132. R. Y. Tsien and T. J. Rink, *in* "Current Methods in Cellular Neurobiology" (J. L. Barber, ed.). Wiley, New York, 1982.
133. F. Di Virgilio, D. P. Lew, and T. Pozzan, *Nature (London)* **310,** 691–693 (1984).
134. B. Dewald, U. Bretz, and M. Baggiolini, *J. Clin. Invest.* **70,** 518–525 (1982).
135. D. G. Wright and J. I. Gallin, *J. Immunol.* **123,** 258–294 (1979).
136. D. G. Wright, D. A. Bralove, and J. I. Gallin, *Am. J. Pathol.* **87,** 273–281 (1977).
137. D. P. Lew, T. Andersson, J. Hed, F. Di Virgilio, T. Pozzan, and O. Stendahl, *Nature (London)* **315,** 509–511 (1985).
138. S. H. Zigmond, J. L. Slonczewski, M. W. Wilde, and M. Carson, *Cell Motil. Cytoskeleton* **9,** 184–189 (1988).
139. F. S. Southwick, G. A. Dabiri, M. Paschetto, and S. H. Zigmond, *J. Cell Biol.* **109,** 156–159 (1989).
140. P. W. Marks and F. R. Maxfield, *J. Cell Biol.* **110,** 43–52 (1990).

CHAPTER 6

Inositol Phosphate Metabolism

Theodora S. Ross

Division of Hematology–Oncology
Washington University School of Medicine
St. Louis, Missouri 63110

Introduction to Phosphatidylinositol Turnover

Phosphatidylinositols are a group of phospholipids which compose up to 10% of the lipid of eukaryotic cells. These lipids are the precursors for the water-soluble inositol phosphates, many of which are putative messenger molecules. Following the original observation that cholinergic stimulation of pancreatic slices results in an increased incorporation of $^{32}PO_4$ into phosphatidylinositol (1–3), rapid turnover of phosphatidylinositols has been observed in many cells in response to a variety of agonists (4).

This "phosphatidylinositol effect" has subsequently been shown to yield at lease three types of signaling molecules: inositol phosphates, diacylglycerol, and arachidonic acid. The inositol phosphates are likely to bear several messages and are the focus of this chapter. Diacylglycerol activates protein kinase C (5). Arachidonate, released from diacylglycerol by diacylglycerol lipase, from monoacylglycerol by monoacylglycerol lipase, and from phosphatidylinositol by phospholipase A_2, is a metabolic precursor of eicosanoids such as thromboxane A_2 and prostaglandin I_2 (6).

Cellular and Molecular Mechanisms of Inflammation, Volume 3

Before speculating on the functions of inositol phosphates and discussing how the inositol phosphates are metabolized, the structure of inositol phosphates is described (7). Without a basic understanding of inositol phosphate structure, it is more difficult to appreciate the biological significance of the fact that several inositol phosphates as well as several highly specific enzymes exist in cells. *myo*-Inositol has five equatorial hydroxyls and an axial hydroxyl (position 2 on the inositol ring). If one divides *myo*-inositol with a plane containing the 2- and 5-position hydroxyls, it can be seen that each half is the mirror image of the other; that is, the *myo*-inositol molecule is nonchiral, as are inositol phosphates containing phosphates substituted at the 2 or 5 position (Fig. 1). *myo*-Inositols substitutes with a phosphate at the 1, 3, 4, or 6 position convert to a chiral or asymmetric molecule, specified as D- or L-inositol monophosphates. *myo*-Inositol 1-phosphate derived from phosphatidylinositol isolated from mammalian cells is of the D configuration (8). Because of this, all of the inositol phosphates derived from these lipids are assumed to have the D configuration.

Discovering the Biological Role of Inositol Phosphates

Phosphatidylinositol-specific phospholipase C (PLC) catalyzes the hydrolysis of phosphatidylinositols to produce directly or indirectly the poly- and monophosphorylated inositols (Fig. 2). Some of these inositol phosphates have been studied extensively as putative second messengers, and the metabolisms of most of these molecules have been elucidated (9–13). Ins(1,4,5)P_3 promotes Ca^{2+} release from internal stores and is the only in-

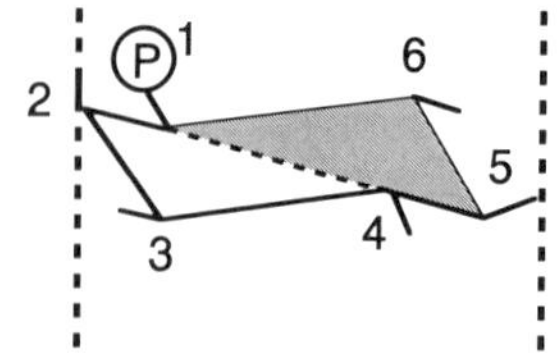

FIGURE 1

Structure of D-*myo*-inositol 1-phosphate.

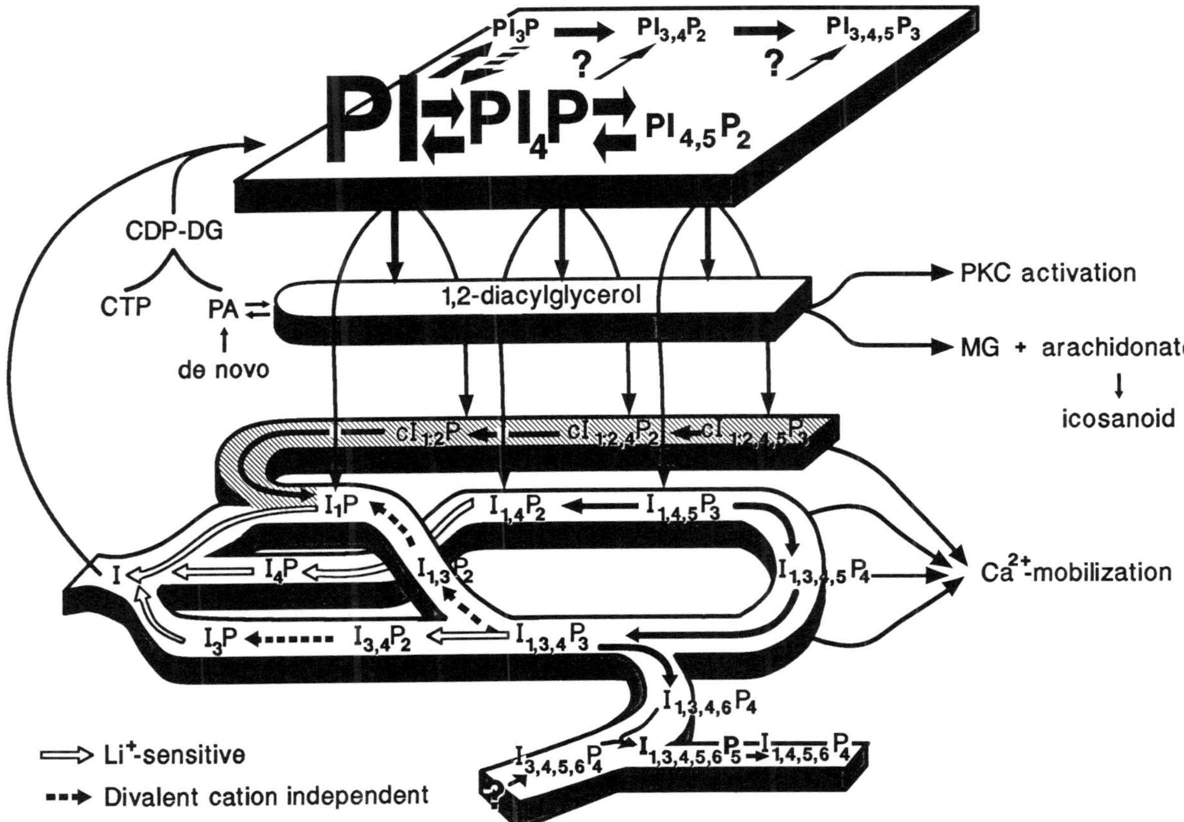

FIGURE 2

Pathways of inositol phosphate metabolism. PKC, Protein kinase C; MG, monoacylglycerol; DG, diacylglycerol; PA, phosphatidate.

ositol phosphate with a function that is widely documented and accepted. The discovery of Ins(1,4,5)P_3 as the mediator of intracellular Ca^{2+} release is well reviewed. However, the steps involved in making the discovery are valuable to review whenever one begins to evaluate the putative functions of other inositol phosphates.

Initially, a correlation between agonist-stimulated Ca^{2+} mobilization and "phosphatidylinositol turnover" was established (14, 15). It was then determined in several cell lines that the rapid release of Ca^{2+} correlated with a concomitant elevation of intracellular Ins(1,4,5)P_3 levels. It was hypothesized that the Ins(1,4,5)P_3 somehow mediated the Ca^{2+} release. This idea was tested *in vitro* by adding Ins(1,4,5)P_3 to $^{45}Ca^{2+}$-loaded microsomal fractions (16–18) or $^{45}Ca^{2+}$-loaded permeabilized cells (19–23). Release of the $^{45}Ca^{2+}$ was demonstrated, and the kinetics of release were consistent with the rate of Ca^{2+} mobilization in intact cells. This response to Ins(1,4,5)P_3 was shown to be saturable and had K_m values in the range of the agonist-stimulated cellular response (20). The Ca^{2+} release was shown to be specific in that other inositol phosphates were either much less potent or ineffective (21). Finally, a specific receptor for Ins(1,4,5)P_3 was identified (24–28), characterized (29–31), purified (32), cloned (33–36), and reconstituted into lipid vesicles to enhance Ins(1,4,5)P_3-mediated calcium flux (37, 38).

The complexity of the metabolism of inositol phosphates suggests that inositol phosphates, in addition to Ins(1,4,5)P_3, which is only one of at least 20 different inositol phosphates isolated from cells, also bear messages. Several functions for these molecules have been proposed, but most of these are at the correlation level of the discovery process. These correlations are reviewed during discussions of the enzymes which form and degrade the particular inositol phosphates.

Many of the enzymes which create this complex metabolism have been purified, characterized, and cloned. Further progress in elucidating the biological roles of these molecules lies in purifying and cloning the remaining enzymes. The cDNAs can be used to manipulate the levels of these enzymes in hopes of identifying and characterizing biological phenomena which result from the alteration of the cellular concentrations of the inositol phosphates. Although the PLC enzymes and the pathways of interconversion of phosphatidylinositols via phosphorylation and dephosphorylation at the 3, 4, and 5 positions are not the topic of this review, they are discussed briefly in order to place them in the context of inositol phosphate metabolism. Focus is then shifted to the metabolism, function, and regulation of the water-soluble inositol phosphates.

Interconversion of the Phosphatidylinositols

PtdIns and PtdIns phosphates are interconverted by a series of kinases and phosphatases (upper panel of Fig. 2). The recent discoveries of these metabolic pathways are reminiscent of the complexity of the metabolism of water-soluble inositol phosphates. PtdIns(4)P and PtdIns(4,5)P_2, which represent approximately 0.1% of the total cellular lipid, are synthesized sequentially by 4- and 5-position-specific kinases, respectively (39). These two lipids can also be phosphorylated at the 3 position. There are two types of PtdIns kinases: 3 position specific (type I) and 4 position specific (type II). There are also isoforms of each of these types (for a comprehensive review see Ref. 40). A PtdIns(4)P 5-kinase has been purified from human red blood cell membranes (41) and is relatively specific for PtdIns(4)P in that it phosphorylates PtdIns(4)P with a 100-fold higher velocity than PtdIns. The phosphomonoesterases which catalyze the removal of the phosphates have not been extensively characterized (42).

The PtdIns lipids phosphorylated in the 3 position are a very popular topic to study, since the PtdIns 3-kinase has been shown to associate with several growth factor receptors (43, 44), oncogene products (45, 46), and the polyoma middle T antigen–pp60$^{c\text{-}src}$ complex (47), suggesting that PtdIns(3)P is involved in cell proliferation. Using antiphosphotyrosine antibodies, Auger *et al.* (48) found that immunoprecipitates have PtdIns 3-kinase activity that utilizes all of the "traditional" inositol lipids as substrates. Whether this pathway occurs *in vivo* is not known (Fig. 2, questionable arrows in the top panel). PLC does not cleave the 3-phosphate-containing lipids (49, 50). PtdIns(3)P is metabolized by the action of a 3-phosphomonoesterase activity that appears to be the same enzyme which specifically catalyzes the hydrolysis of the 3-phosphate from Ins(1,3)P_2: inositol polyphosphate 3-phosphatase (see below for a discussion of the 3-phosphatase; see also Ref. 51).

These 3-phosphate-containing lipids have been isolated from platelets (52–54). Using the specific inositol phosphate phosphatases (described below), we have been able to definitively identify the 3-phosphate-containing inositol lipids in platelets and NIH-3T3 cells and determine the major pathway for formation of these lipids. PtdIns(3,4)P_2 and PtdIns(3,4,5)P_3 have two possible sources (Fig. 2). It was found that the pathway involving 4-and 5-kinase-catalyzed reactions is the major pathway. This route was discovered when cells were labeled with $^{32}PO_4$ and the

3-phosphate-containing inositol lipids were analyzed prior to equilibrium. After deacylation and deglyceration the specific enzymes were used to determine which phosphate on each lipid had the highest specific activity. This phosphate is the last phosphate added during *in vivo* synthesis (52, 55).

PtdIns 3-kinase

The PtdIns 3-kinase (type I PtdIns kinase) has recently been purified (56, 57) and has at least two isoforms: Type I has a mass of 110 kDa both by gel filtration and Sodium dodecyl sulfate–polyacrylamide gel electrophoresis (SDS–PAGE) analysis; type II has a mass of 190 kDa upon gel filtration analysis and consists of 85- and 110-kDa subunits, as estimated by SDS–PAGE analysis. These data suggest that the 110-kDa subunit is the catalytic subunit. The 85-kDa subunit has been cloned and the primary structure encodes *src* homology domains, designated SH2, which are found in several of the proteins that associate with oncogene products and activated growth factor receptors (58). Consistent with the presence of this sequence, it has been demonstrated, with a ligand blot, that the polyoma middle T protein associates with the 85-kDa subunit (56).

Since these lipids are of very low concentrations in the cell and PLC does not catalyze their hydrolysis, they are not likely to be a significant source of diacylglycerol and the presently known inositol phosphates of the cell. They may function as lipids or as precursors of novel messenger molecules. A correlation of the PtdIns(3,4)P_2 levels with actin polymerization (59) has been observed, suggesting that these molecules anchor actin filaments to the membrane. As with the water-soluble inositol phosphates, the inositol phospholipid pathway is becoming very complex. The future discoveries of additional kinases and phosphatases and their regulation may indicate how these lipids are linked to cellular functions.

Production of Inositol Phosphates

The enzymatic reactions catalyzed by specific enzymes of the PtdIns cycle are listed in Table I. The primary structures of several PLC enzymes, the inositol monophosphatase, inositol cyclic 1:2-phosphate 2-phosphohydrolase (cyclic hydrolase), Ins(1,4,5)P_3 3-kinase (3-kinase), inositol polyphosphate 1-phosphatase (1-phosphatase), and one of the inositol poly-

TABLE I

Enzymes of Inositol Phosphate Metabolism

Enzyme	Substrate
PLC	PtdIns, PtdIns(4)P, PtdIns(4,5)P_2
Monophosphatase	Ins(1)P, Ins(4)P, Ins(5)P
Cyclic hydrolase	GroPIns, cIns(1:2)P
3-Kinase	Ins(1,4,5)P_3
1-Phosphatase	Ins(1,4)P_2, Ins(1,3,4)P_3
5-Phosphatase	cIns(1,4,5)P_3, Ins(1,4,5)P_3, Ins(1,3,4,5)P_4
3-Phosphatase	Ins(1,3)P_2, PtdIns(3)P
4-Phosphatase	Ins(3,4)P_2, Ins(1,3,4)P_3
cIns(1:2,4)P_2 4-phosphatase	cIns(1:2,4)P_2
6-Kinase	Ins(1,3,4)P_3
1-Kinase	Ins(3,4,5,6)P_4
5-Kinase	Ins(1,3,4,6)P_4

phosphate 5-phosphatases (5-phosphatase) are known. The inositol polyphosphate 3-phosphatase (3-phosphatase), inositol polyphosphate 4-phosphatase (4-phosphatase), cIns(1:2,4)P_2 4-phosphatase, 6-kinase, 1-kinase, and 5-kinase enzymes have not yet been cloned.

PtdIns-Specific PLC

PLC catalyzes the reactions shown in Fig. 3. This figure illustrates that six different inositol phosphates are formed, depending on the substrate and conditions of the reaction. Recently, it was shown that both the cyclic and noncyclic products are sterically inverted at the phosphorus (60). This is a significant observation because it demonstrates that the mechanism of this reaction involves a direct nucleophilic attack of the phosphodiester bond by either water or the 2-hydroxyl. If the cyclic product were merely an intermediate of the reaction, it would have a configuration opposite that of the noncyclic product.

Guanine nucleotides activate PLC activity when added to membrane preparations. Recently, a GTP-binding protein specifically linked to PLC-β activation has been identified (G_q). This activation is due to an increase in intrinsic specific activity of PLC-β as well as a decreased requirement of the reaction for Ca^{2+} (61). Another characteristic of PLC is that there are several

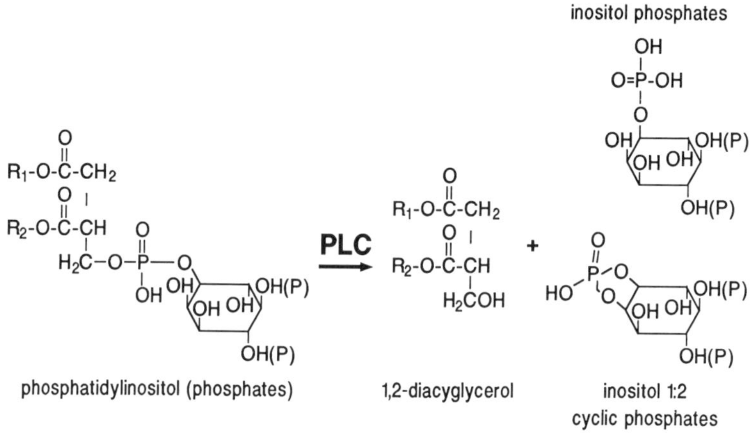

FIGURE 3

Reaction catalyzed by phospholipase C (PLC).

isoforms of PLC; the members of this family have been reviewed (62–64). The existence of several forms may be due to a needed redundancy for protection against mutations which, without this redundancy, would be lethal. However, it also seems likely that the different forms carry out distinct biological functions. In other words, the PLC-catalyzed reaction is central to a signal transduction pathway in which fine tuning of this reaction is needed. This may be accomplished with different G proteins or by the use of isoenzymes with different properties for different responses to agonist stimulation. This phenomenon of multiple enzyme forms in the same cell appears again when another reaction central to this signal transduction system, the 5-phosphatase "signal-terminating" enzyme reaction, is discussed.

The γ isoform of PLC has received much attention due to several interesting observations. Two isoforms of this γ subtype have been cloned (62, 65, 66). In addition to having the conserved catalytic domains (65), these γ PLCs have the *src* homology (SH2) domains described previously for the 85-kDa subunit of the type II PtdIns 3-kinase (67, 68). As predicted, PLC-γ also associates with the epidermal growth factor (EGF) and platelet-derived growth factor (PDGF) receptors and is phosphorylated on tyrosine in response to growth factors. The other types of PLC have not been shown to be phosphorylated on tyrosine. This phosphorylation activates PLC (69) and correlates with the association of PLC with the PDGF and EGF receptors (70–73).

Stable overexpression of PLC-γ in NIH-3T3 cells results in elevated inositol phosphate levels in response to PDGF stimulation, but does not alter the magnitude of the growth response (increase of [^{3}H]thymidine incorporation) to PDGF (63, 74). This suggests that either PLC-γ expression and PtdIns turnover are unnecessary for the normal response to growth factors or that the cells have a way of adapting to altered PtdIns turnover. Unfortunately, other enzymatic activities of the PtdIns pathway have not yet been assayed in these stable PLC-γ-transfected cell lines. Alteration of these activities upon PLC overexpression may give clues as to possible secondary effects of PLC-γ overexpression. Adaptation to this overexpression is a likely explanation of the lack of an effect on cell growth, since injection of PLC into NIH-3T3 cells does lead to increased [^{3}H]thymidine incorporation, a marker of cell division (75), and serum-stimulated DNA synthesis is inhibited by injection of PLC antibodies into cells (76). It is possible that the different PLCs are linked to different cellular functions [e.g., PLC-γ with growth and PLC-β with vision (77)].

Cyclic Inositol Phosphate Pathway

The cyclic inositol phosphate pathway (Fig. 2, shaded pathway) is often ignored in reviews of inositol phosphate metabolism. Despite this, the potential for discovery of cyclic inositol phosphate functions remains very high due to several recent findings, outlined below.

Possible functions for cIns(1:2,4,5)P_3 are the alteration of membrane conductances in *Limulus* photoreceptor cells (78) and *Xenopus* oocytes (79) and the mobilization of intracellular calcium stores (78, 80, 81). The ratio of cyclic to noncyclic inositol phosphates in the cell increases with the duration of agonist stimulation (82, 83). This may be due to a lower rate of turnover of the cyclic inositol phosphates, but the significance of this ratio is not known. The ratio produced *in vitro* by PLC-mediated cleavage of phosphatidylinositols increases when PtdIns is the substrate, rather than PtdIns(4)P or PtdIns(4,5)P_2; when the pH of the reaction is lowered to 5.5 from 7.0; when calcium is increased; or when PLC-β is used as a catalyst, rather than the 100 or γ isoform of PLC (84).

Most of the cyclic inositol phosphate in the cell is in the form of cIns(1:2)P. cIns(1:2)P is derived both directly from the degradation of PtdIns by PLC and indirectly from PLC degradation of PtdIns(4,5)P_2 and PtdIns(4)P followed by dephosphorylation of cIns(1:2,4,5)P_3 to cIns(1:2,4)P_2 and dephosphorylation of cIns(1:2,4)P_2 to cIns(1:2)P. The inositol polyphosphate 5-phosphatase hydrolyzes cIns(1:2,4,5)P_3 to cIns(1,4)P_2, but has a very poor affinity compared to noncyclic Ins(1,4,5)P_3 (85). This may explain why cIns(1:2,4,5)P_3 returns to basal levels at a slower rate than Ins(1,4,5)P_3 in agonist-stimulated cells. A cIns(1:2,4)P_2 4-phosphatase from bovine brain extracts converts cIns(1:2,4)P_2 to cIns(1:2)P (V. S. Bansal and P. W. Majerus, unpublished observations). This is likely to be different from the inositol polyphosphate 4-phosphatase (86), since it requires Mg^{2+} for catalytic activity. The protein which catalyzes the hydrolysis of the cyclic bond, cyclic hydrolase, does not recognize the polyphosphorylted cyclic inositol phosphates (87) and is likely to be a rate-limiting enzyme of this pathway, since as it catalyzes the only reaction known to cleave the cyclic bond. This enzyme has several interesting properties, which are outlined below.

Cyclic Hydrolase

The primary sequence of the cyclic hydrolase is identical to that of lipocortin III, a member of a large family of homologous calcium- and phospholipid-binding proteins without defined biological functions (88). Some of these proteins have been shown to be phosphorylated in response to growth factors. The purified enzyme (33 kDa) is inhibited by inositol 2-phosphate [Ins(2)P], Zn^{2+}, and glycerophosphoinositol (GroPIns) and stimulated by acidic phospholipids (87, 89). The pattern of interaction with particular phospholipids is the same as that previously observed for lipocortins (88, 90). The mechanism of inhibition by GroPIns is due to its ability to act as a substrate for this enzyme (89). The regulatory significance of this reaction is unclear, as the level of GroPIns-hydrolyzing activity measured in cellular extracts does not inversely correlate with the cellular levels of GroPIns (T. S. Ross and P. W. Majerus, unpublished observations). The presence of significant amounts of Ins(2)P and GroPIns in cells has been well documented (89, 91) and suggests that they may function as regulators of cellular cIns(1:2)P levels.

Measurement of the cyclic hydrolase activity in cellular extracts has unveiled a very interesting pattern. Cells with relatively low to nondetectable activity were either completely transformed or partially transformed (92). When levels of cyclic inositol phosphates were measured in these cells, it was found that cIns(1:2)P increased in proportion to the decreased cyclic hydrolase activity. The enzyme activity is also increased within one cell type when it is in a confluent state as compared to a logarithmically growing state. Overexpression of cyclic hydrolase in cells decreases the cIns(1:2)P levels as well as the final saturation density. In addition, high endogenous expression of cyclic hydrolase in cells tends to correlate with the differentiated state (e.g., high levels in platelets, brain, and neutrophils and low levels in several immortalized tissue culture cell lines of fibroblasts and T cells). The finding that this correlation exists both in nature and during heterologous expression of the enzyme makes the discovery of a cellular function for cIns(1:2)P likely to be successful. Further studies of the regulation of the cyclic hydrolase activity and cIns(1:2)P cellular levels will yield valuable information as to how to continue the quest for the function(s) of the cyclic bond.

Ins(1,4,5)P_3/Ins(1,3,4,5)P_4 Pathway

It was originally thought that all of the InsP_3 in the cell was the Ins (1,4,5)P_3 isomer. However, subsequent studies have demonstrated that the Ins(1,3,4)P_3 isomer was also formed in cells (93). This led to the delineation of the "tris/tetrakisphosphate pathway." The discovery of this pathway involved examination of the kinetics of the agonist-stimulated formation of the InsP_3 isomers (94, 95). It was found that Ins(1,4,5)P_3 increased rapidly in agonist-stimulated cells and that Ins(1,3,4)P_3 levels increased only after a lag time. The origin of Ins(1,3,4)P_3 was a mystery. Possibilities included PLC hydrolysis of a putative PtdIns(3,4)P_2 or isomerization of Ins(1,4,5)P_3. At the time, PtdIns(3,4)P_2 was not found in cells, and the amount of Ins(1,3,4)P_3 was often greater than that of Ins(1,4,5)P_3. This suggested that isomerization of Ins(1,4,5)P_3 was the likely mechanism of the formation of Ins(1,3,4)P_3. It was next demonstrated that Ins(1,3,4,5)P_4 existed in cells (96) and that this IP_4 could be converted when incubated with various cell extracts to Ins(1,3,4)P_3 (97–99). Irvine *et al.* (100) subsequently identified a 3-kinase activity in cell extracts. This isomerization pathway is:

$$\text{Ins}(1,4,5)P_3 \xrightarrow{\text{3-kinase}} \text{Ins}(1,3,4,5)P_4 \xrightarrow{\text{5-phosphatase}} \text{Ins}(1,3,4)P_3$$

Ins(1,4,5)P_3 is the most well studied of the noncyclic inositol phosphates. Figure 2 shows that it has two possible fates: As described above, it is either phosphorylated to Ins(1,3,4,5)P_4 or dephosphorylated to Ins(1,4)P_2. The enzymes that catalyze these conversions are 3-kinase and 5-phosphatase, respectively. 5-Phosphatase is considered a signal-terminating enzyme, whereas 3-kinase is likely to be a signal-terminating as well as signal-producing enzyme. Ins(1,4,5)P_3 3-kinase does not metabolize cIns(1:2,4,5)P_3 (86), whereas 5-phosphatase does (86). The affinity of the kinase for Ins(1,4,5)P_3 (K_m = 0.2 μM) makes it a possible competitor of 5-phosphatase (K_m = 5 μM) for utilizing the Ins(1,4,5)P_3 in the cell.

Possible Functions of Ins(1,3,4,5)P_4

The best evidence in favor of Ins(1,3,4,5)P_4's having a messenger molecule function is the demonstration by Theibert *et al.* (101) that specific Ins (1,3,4,5)P_4 membrane binding sites in rat brain can be solubilized and separated from Ins(1,4,5)P_3 binding sites. Prior to this observation, there had been studies indicating that Ins(1,3,4,5)P_4 somehow functions in modulating intracellular Ca^{2+} levels. For example, when acetylcholine binds to muscarinic receptors of exocrine acinar cells, cytosolic Ca^{2+} rises, and this activates calcium-dependent K^+ channels (102). If one injects Ins(1,4,5)P_3 and Ins(1,3,4,5)P_4 simultaneously, one can mimic this response. Injection of either of these inositol phosphates alone has no effect. It has been suggested that Ins(1,4,5)P_3 mobilizes intracellular sources of calcium and Ins(1,3,4,5)P_4 controls entry from the extracellular fluid in concert with Ins(1,4,5)P_3 (10). However, there is a paucity of data supporting this hypothesis, and the original studies which were the basis for the formation of this hypothesis have not been reproducible (103). There should be less speculation about calcium mobilization and more investigation of Ins(1,3,4,5)P_4 as a signal for other biological events in addition to Ca^{2+} mobilization. For example, decreasing the expression of 5-phosphatase would be expected to cause a build-up of Ins(1,3,4,5)P_4 in the cell, whereas decreasing the expression of 3-kinase would indicate how Ins(1,3,4,5)P_4 deficiency effects the phenotype of the cell.

Ins(1,4,5)P_3 3-kinase

As one would expect of a reaction which converts one messenger molecule [Ins(1,4,5)P_3] to another [Ins(1,3,4,5)P_4], the 3-kinase enzyme is highly regulated. Examples of its regulation in cells includes 14-fold increases of activity during development from fetus to adult (104), activation by calcium and calmodulin (101, 105–109), and 7-fold increased specific activity in *src*-transformed cells (110). The primary structure of the enzyme (111) has several PEST sequences and a calmodulin binding domain. It has been proposed that correlation of PEST sequences (single-letter amino acid code) and sensitivity to the calpain protease or calmodulin activation is due to negatively charged amino acids' binding calcium, which then binds both calpain and calmodulin locally. Purification of this enzyme in the presence of a specific calpain inhibitor increases yields and decreases the 3-kinase-immunoreactive bands from seven to three in purified preparations stained with anti-3-kinase monoclonal antibodies. Although this indicates that this cleavage occurs during purification, it may be a route for regulating 3-kinase activity in intact cells.

Transient expression of 3-kinase has been successful in COS cells (111). However, the phenotypic results of overexpression have not yet been reported. Expression of mutants of 3-kinase which have deleted PEST sites may answer the question as to which PEST sites are important for modulation of activity. In addition there is a protein kinase A consensus sequence near the N terminus of the second PEST region which may also contribute to modulation of the enzyme activity in cells. For example, in hepatocytes 3-kinase activity is stimulated by a combination of protein kinase A and protein kinase C activation (112). Coexpression of 3-kinase with 5-phosphatase, which recognizes both the substrate and the product of 3-kinase, may give a spectrum of phenotypes and Ins(1,3,4,5)P_4/Ins(1,4,5)P_3 ratios. It will be interesting to determine whether these levels correlate inversely with these activities, as was found with cyclic hydrolase (see above).

Inositol Polyphosphate 5-phosphatase

The 5-phosphatase has three known inositol phosphate substrates: Ins(1,4,5)P_3, cIns(1:2,4,5)P_3, and Ins(1,3,4,5)P_4. Since these are all putative signaling molecules, as described above, this enzyme is signal terminating, and therefore it is likely to be tightly regulated. An example of this regulation has been observed in phorbol ester-treated platelets (113). 5-Phosphatase activity has been detected in all cells tested and is composed of more than one form distributed both in cytosol and in membranes. This is reminiscent of the presence of several phospholipase C isoforms (62, 63). Two 5-phosphatase types have been identified from human platelets (114, 115), rat brain (116, 117), and bovine brain (118). The two types from platelets have been purified, and type II has been cloned (119). The reported affinities of these enzymes for Ins(1,3,4,5)$P_{4)}$ and Ins(1,4,5)P_3 vary (for a comprehensive review see Ref. 120), and in general the 5-phosphatase isoforms have higher affinities for Ins(1,3,4,5)P_4 than for Ins(1,4,5)P_3. A membrane-bound 5-phosphatase has been partially purified and has properties similar to type I (117). Finally, the platelet type I 5-phosphatase is phosphorylated and activated by protein kinase C (121).

The primary sequence of the type II platelet enzyme has several consensus sequences for different protein kinases and has a predicted molecular mass of 75 kDa. An antibody directed against either the N terminus or C region of recombinant protein precipitates type II, but not type I, activity. This result indicates that the type I and II activities are immunologically distinct as well as physically distinct, as evidenced by their different chromatographic properties (119). With the acquisition of this clone and antibodies which immunoprecipitate and blot the enzyme, the cloning of the other isoforms and study of their regulation *in vivo* are events of the near future.

Other Pathways of Inositol Phosphate Metabolism

The inositol polyphosphate 1-phosphatase catalyzes the hydrolysis of Ins(1,3,4)P_3 and Ins(1,4)P_2 at the 1-position phosphate (122). The latter two inositol phosphates have not been found to have convincing functions in any physiological system. However, some measured effects of these inositol phosphatase include Ins(1,4)P_2 activation of human DNA polymerase α (123) and Ins(1,3,4)P_3-mediated calcium mobilization in Swiss mouse 3T3 cells (EC_{50} of 10 μM) (80). This calcium-mobilizing activity is plausible, as the cellular concentration of Ins(1,3,4)P_3 has been shown to reach 25 μM levels in stimulated cells. It has been suggested that Ins(1,3,4)P_3 functions to deplete intracellular stores of calcium as a mechanism of desensitization of cells to chronically elevated levels of Ins(1,4,5)P_3. Unfortunately, these calcium-mobilizing data have not been followed with receptor isolation, cloning, and reconstitution, as in the Ins(1,4,5)P_3 case. At present there is little evidence for a cellular function of Ins(1,3,4)P_3. If it is true that Ins(1,3,4)P_3 has little biological significance, why is the metabolism of this inositol trisphosphate so complex? Why does its metabolism vary between tissues? Is it possible that this tissue-specific complexity reflects the importance of one of its products? The answer to these questions may be obtained by manipulating the metabolism of Ins(1,3,4)P_3 with molecular genetic techniques. Of the enzymes which metabolize Ins(1,3,4)P_3, only the 1-phosphatase has been cloned.

Inositol Polyphosphate 1-phosphatase

The mass of the 1-phosphatase is 44 kDa, as determined by SDS–PAGE (124, 125) as well as predicted from the cDNA (126). It is likely that there is only one form of this enzyme, since rabbit antiserum, prepared against homogeneous protein purified from bovine brain, precipitates more than 95% of the activity which hydrolyzes Ins(1,4)P_2 to Ins(4)P in several tissues (127). As is described for the monophosphatase, Li^+ inhibits this enzyme noncompetitively, with k_i values of 0.3 and 6 m*M* for Ins(1,3,4)P_3 and Ins(1,4)P_2 hydrolyses, respectively (124, 127). Unexpectedly, the primary structure of this enzyme (13) has very little, if any, homology with the monophosphatase (see below), in spite of the fact that they are both noncompetitively inhibited by Li^+. The overexpression of this enzyme in cells is likely to yield a very interesting result, since the Ins(1,3,4)P_3 substrate is at a three-way branching of inositol phosphate metabolism (Fig. 2). Changing the directions may give clues as to the function of either Ins(1,3,4)P_3 itself or the inositol phosphate products resulting from its metabolism.

Inositol Polyphosphate 4-phosphatase

Ins(1,3,4)P_3 is converted to Ins(1,3)P_2 by a specific 4-phosphatase which is metal ion independent (128). This enzyme has been partially purified from the soluble fraction of calf brain (86) and has been found to have a mass of 110 kDa, as estimated by both gel filtration and SDS-PAGE. The 4-phosphatase also degrades Ins(3,4)P_2 to Ins(3)P. The ratio of 4-phosphatase to 1-phosphatase activity in a variety of cell types has been determined (127), and only in the brain does the 4-phosphatase activity predominate. Other than the latter observation, the role of this enzyme in the biology of inositol phosphates has not yet been investigated.

Inositol Polyphosphate 3-phosphatase

The Ins(1,3)P_2 produced by the 4-phosphatase-mediated hydrolysis of Ins(1,3,4)P_3 is metabolized by a specific 3-phosphatase that does not require metal ions for activity (128). This enzyme has recently been purified to homogeneity and has some very interesting properties (51). As mentioned in the discussion of PtdIns(3)P metabolism, this enzyme also uses PtdIns(3)P as a substrate. In addition it has been isolated in two forms: Type I is 65 kDa by SDS–PAGE analysis and 110 kDa by gel filtration; type II is 147 kDa by gel filtration and consists of two subunits of 65 and 78 kDa, as demonstrated by SDS–PAGE. The 65-kDa subunit of each type is either the same or highly related to the 65-kDa subunit of the other 3-phosphatase isoform. The type I enzyme prefers the water-soluble substrate [Ins(1,3)P_2], and the type II prefers the lipid-soluble substrate [PtdIns(3)P]. This pattern of two isoforms which share a similar subunit is reminiscent of the two forms of PtdIns 3-kinase described earlier. It may not be coincidental that both of these activities mediate the modification of the 3 position on the inositol ring of phosphatidylinositol. It is likely that the cloning of these two enzymes will demonstrate some interesting homologies.

Phosphorylation of Ins(1,3,4)P_3

Ins(1,3,4)P_3 can be phosphorylated by a 6-kinase, yielding Ins(1,3,4,6)P_4 (120, 130–132). Since this reaction requires energy, it is very possible that this conversion of Ins(1,3,4)P_3 is of physiological significance. Ins(1,3,4,5,6)P_5 is produced from a Ins(1,3,4,6)P_4 5-kinase or a Ins(3,4,5,6)P_4 1-kinase (131). The 6-kinase has been partially purified from liver (13) and brain (132) and has a mass of 30 kDa, as estimated by gel filtration. Interestingly, it is inhibited by 10 μM Ins(1,3,4,5)P_4 (133). Could this inhibition be a biological function for Ins(1,3,4,5)P_4? Is the formation of Ins(1,3,4)P_3 just a part of the route for formation of Ins(1,3,4,6)P_4 or Ins(1,3,4,5,6)P_5? Determination of the primary structure and regulation of the enzyme(s) which catalyzes these reactions may answer these questions.

Monophosphatase

The monophosphatase cDNA has been isolated (134) and has a novel sequence with significant homology with the QAX protein of *Neurospora crassa* and the QUTG protein of *Aspergillus nidulans*, both of which are thought to be involved in quinate metabolism. The relationship of this metabolic pathway and the PtdIns pathway is not clear. The purified protein catalyzes the hydrolytic removal of phosphate groups in the 1, 3, 4, and 5 positions on the inositol ring (124, 135). The latter nonselectivity for a particular position on the inositol ring is anomalous as compared to the more specific inositol polyphosphate phosphatases. This enzyme, like the 1-phosphatase, is inhibited noncompetitively by Li^+. Li^+ traps the enzyme in an inositol phosphate–enzyme complex which prevents hydrolysis of the product (136, 137). With this inhibition in mind, it is tempting to speculate that the clinically useful effects of Li^+ in treating various mental disorders is due to a mechanism involving the monophosphatase and/or the 1-phosphatase (for a review see Ref. 138). The results of underexpression of the cDNA (using either antisense techniques or overexpression of inactive subunits) can be predicted to be similar to the effects of Li^+ on cells which include increased inositol phosphates, diminished elevation of Ins(1,4,5)P_3 and Ins(1,3,4,5)P_4 upon agonist stimulation (consistent with the inositol depletion hypothesis), and altered development (i.e., teratogenesis). However, Li^+ is much less selective, and some of its effects may not be specific to monophosphatase inhibition. Although overexpression of the cDNA clone has not yet been reported, it is not expected to biologically affect the cell, as the monophosphatase is not known to be a rate-limiting enzyme because it has several substrates which represent the convergence of at least six different metabolic pathways (Fig. 2). Also, the enzyme activity has not been found to be altered in different cell types, at different stages of cell growth, or in response to cell stimulation.

Closing Comments

A review of the recent findings and ideas about phosphatidylinositol metabolism with reference to the previously established facts unveils many details that do not yet fit into these new stories. From this overview it is clear that the molecular genetic strategy for studying the key reactions of inositol phosphate metabolism and inositol phosphate functions is making progress. However, it is disappointing that the sequences of the presently isolated clones share little homology. One might have predicted that there would be a common inositol-binding sequence in all of the enzymes that mediate the different pathways of Fig. 2. Finally, the continued search for new regulatory proteins that bind and/or metabolize these inositol phosphates is a route of study which, as in the past, will be both surprising and exciting.

Acknowledgments

This research was supported by National Heart, Lung and Blood Institute grants HLBI 14147 (to the Specialized Center for Research in Thrombosis) and HLBI 16634 and by the Monsanto Corporation (St. Louis, MO) and the Life and Health Insurance Medical Research Fund. I thank Philip Majerus and Kevin Caldwell for critically reading the manuscript.

References

1. M. R. Hokin and L. E. Hokin, *J. Biol. Chem.* **203,** 967–977 (1953).
2. L. E. Hokin and M. R. Hokin, *Biochim. Biophys. Acta* **21,** 168–170 (1955).
3. L. E. Hokin and M. R. Hokin, *J. Biol. Chem.* **233,** 805–810 (1958).
4. L. E. Hokin, *Annu. Rev. Biochem.* **54,** 205–235 (1985).
5. Y. Nishizuka, *Science* **233,** 305–312 (1986).
6. P. W. Majerus, D. B. Wilson, T. M. Connolly, T. E. Bross, and E. J. Neufeld, *Trends Biochem. Sci.* **10,** 168–171 (1985).
7. R. Parthasarathy and F. Eisenberg, *Biochem. J.* **235,** 313–322 (1986).
8. C. E. Ballou and L. I. Pizer, *J. Am. Chem. Soc.* **82,** 3333–3335 (1960).
9. P. W. Majerus, T. M. Connolly, V. S. Bansal, R. C. Inhorn, T.S. Ross, and D. L. Lips, *J. Biol. Chem.* **263,** 3051–3054 (1988).
10. R. F. Irvine, R. M. Moor, W. K. Pollock, P. M. Smith, and K. A. Wreggett, *Philos. Trans. R. Soc. London, B* **320,** 281–298 (1988).
11. S. B. Shears, *Biochem. J.* **260,** 313–324 (1989).
12. R. S. Rana and L. E. Hokin, *Physiol. Rev.* **70,** 115–162 (1990).
13. V. S. Bansal and P. W. Majerus, *Annu. Rev. Cell Biol.* **6,** 41–67 (1990).
14. R. H. Michell, *Biochim. Biophys. Acta* **415,** 81–147 (1975).
15. R. H. Michell, C. J. Kirk, L. M. Jones, C. P. Downes, and J. A. Creba, *Philos. Trans. R. Soc. London, B* **296,** 123–137 (1981).
16. M. Prentki, T. J. Biden, D. Janjic, R. F. Irvine, M. J. Berridge, and C. B. Wollheim, *Nature (London)* **309,** 562–564 (1984).
17. A. P. Dawson and R. F. Irvine, *Biochem. Biophys. Res. Commun.* **120,** 858–864 (1984).
18. F. A. O'Rourke, S. P. Halenda, G. B. Zavoico, and M. B. Feinstein, *J. Biol. Chem.* **260,** 956–962 (1985).
19. H. Streb, R. F. Irvine, M. J. Berridge, and I. Schulz, *Nature (London)* **306,** 67–69 (1983).
20. S. K. Joseph, A. P. Thomas, R. J. Williams, R. F. Irvine, and J. R. Williamson, *J. Biol. Chem.* **259,** 3077–3081 (1984).
21. G. M. Burgess, R. F. Irvine, M. J. Berridge, J. D. McKinney, and J. W. Putney, *Biochem. J.* **224,** 741–746 (1984).
22. E. Suematsu, M. Hirata, T. Hashimoto, and H. Kuriyama, *Biochem. Biophys. Res. Commun.* **120,** 481–485 (1984).
23. M. C. Gershengorn, E. Geras, V. S. Purrello, and M. J. Rebecchi, *J. Biol. Chem.* **259,** 10675–10681 (1984).
24. A. J. Baukal, G. Guillemette, R. Rubin, A. Spat, and K. J. Catt, *Biochem. Biophys. Res. Commun.* **133,** 532–538 (1985).
25. A. Spat, P. G. Bradford, J. S. McKinney, R. P. Rubin, and J. W. Putney, *Nature (London)* **319,** 514–516 (1986).
26. G. Guillemette, T. Balla, A. J. Baukal, and K. J. Catt, *Proc. Natl. Acad. Sci. U.S.A.* **84,** 8195–8199 (1987).
27. A. Spat, G. L. Lukacs, I. Eberhjardt, L. Kiesel, and B. Runnebaum, *Biochem. J.* **244,** 493–496 (1987).
28. G. Guillemette, T. Balla, A. J. Baukal, A. Spat, and K. J. Catt, *J. Biol. Chem.* **262,** 1010–1015 (1987).
29. P. F. Worley, J. M. Baraban, S. Supattapone, V. S. Wilson, and S. H. Snyder, *J. Biol. Chem.* **262,** 12132–12136 (1987).

30. P. F. Worley, J. M. Baraban, J. S. Colvin, and S. H. Snyder, *Nature (London)* **325,** 159–161 (1987).
31. S. Supattapone, P. F. Worley, J. M. Baraban, and S. H. Snyder, *J. Biol. Chem.* **263,** 1230–1234 (1988).
32. S. Supattapone, S. K. Danoff, A. Theibert, S. K. Joseph, J. Steiner, and S. H. Snyder, *Proc. Natl. Acad. Sci. U.S.A.* **85,** 8747–8750 (1988).
33. D. T. Nordquist, C. A. Kozak, and H. T. Orr, *J. Neurosci.* **12,** 4780–4789 (1988).
34. G. A. Mignery, T. C. Sudhof, K. Takei, and P. D. Camilli, *Nature (London)* **342,** 192–195 (1989).
35. T. Furuichi, S. Yoshikawa, A. Miyawaki, K. Wada, N. Maeda, and K. Mikoshiba, *Nature (London)* **342,** 32–38 (1989).
36. N. Maeda, T. Kawasaki, S. Nakade, N. Yokota, T. Taguchi, M. Kasai, and K. Mikoshiba, *J. Biol. Chem.* **266,** 1109–1116 (1991).
37. C. D. Ferris, R. L. Huganir, S. Supattapone, and S. H. Snyder, *Nature (London)* **342,** 87–89 (1989).
38. C. D. Ferris, R. L. Huganir, and S. H. Snyder, *Proc. Natl. Acad. Sci. U.S.A.* **87,** 2147–2151 (1990).
39. H. Brockerhoff and C. E. Ballou, *J. Biol. Chem.* **237,** 1764–1766 (1962).
40. C. L. Carpenter and L. C. Cantley, *Biochemistry* **29,** 11147–11156 (1990).
41. L. E. Ling, J. T. Schulz, and L. C. Cantley, *J. Biol. Chem.* **264,** 5080–5088 (1989).
42. P. D. Roach and F. B. St. C. Palmer, *Biochim. Biophys. Acta* **661,** 323–333 (1981).
43. S. R. Coughlin, J. A. Escobedo, and L. T. Williams, *Science* **243,** 1191–1194 (1989).
44. L. Varticovski, B. Drucker, D. Morrison, L. Cantley, and T. Roberts, *Nature (London)* **342,** 699–702 (1989).
45. M. Whitman, C. P. Downes, M. Keeler, T. Keller, and L. Cantley, *Nature (London)* **332,** 644–646 (1988).
46. Y. Fukui, S. Kornbluth, S.-M. Jong, L.-H. Wang, and H. Hanafusa, *Oncogene Res.* **4,** 283–292 (1989).
47. M. Whitman, D. R. Kaplan, B. Schaffhausen, L. Cantley, and T. M. Roberts, *Nature (London)* **315,** 239–242 (1985).
48. K. R. Auger, L. A. Serunian, S. P. Soltoff, P. Libby, and L. C. Cantley, *Cell* **57,** 167–175 (1989).
49. L. A. Serunian, M. T. Haber, T. Fukui, J. W. Kim, S. G. Rhee, J. M. Lowenstein, and L. C. Cantley, *J. Biol. Chem.* **264,** 17809–17815 (1989).
50. D. L. Lips, P. W. Majerus, F. R. Gorga, A. T. Young, and T. L. Benjamin, *J. Biol. Chem.* **264,** 8759–8763 (1989).
51. D. L. Lips, K. K. Caldwell, and P. W. Majerus, *J. Biol. Chem.* **266,** 18378–18386 (1991).
52. T. W. Cunningham, D. L. Lips, V. S. Bansal, K. K. Caldwell, C. A. Mitchell, and P. W. Majerus, *J. Biol. Chem.* **265,** 21676–21683 (1990).
53. G. L. Kucera and S. E. Rittenhouse, *J. Biol. Chem.* **265,** 5345–5348 (1990).
54. R. D. Nolan and E. G. Lapetina, *J. Biol. Chem.* **265,** 2441–2445 (1990).
55. T. C. Cunningham and P. W. Majerus, *Biochem. Biophys. Res.* **175,** 568–576 (1991).
56. C. L. Carpenter, B. C. Duckworth, K. R. Auger, B. Cohen, B. S. Schaffhausen, and L. C. Cantley, *J. Biol. Chem.* **265,** 19704–19711 (1990).
57. F. Shibasaki, Y. Homma, and T. Takenawa, *J. Biol. Chem.* **266,** 10367–10374 (1991).
58. L. C. Cantley, K. R. Auger, C. Carpenter, B. Duckworth, A. Graziani, R. Kapeller, and S. Soltoff, *Cell* **64,** 281–302 (1991).
59. M. Eberle, A. E. Traynor-Kaplan, L. A. Sklar, and J. Norgauer, *J. Biol. Chem.* **265,** 16725–16728 (1990).
60. G. Lin, C. F. Bennet, and M.-D. Tsai, *Biochemistry* **29,** 2747–2757 (1990).

61. A. V. Smrcka, J. R. Hepler, K. O. Brown, and P. C. Sternweis, *Science* **251,** 804–807 (1991).
62. S. G. Rhee, P.-G. Suh, S.-H. Ryu, and S. Y. Lee, *Science* **244,** 546–550 (1989).
63. R. Kriz, L.-L. Linn, L. Sultzman, C. Ellis, C. H. Heldin, T. Pawson, and J. Knopf, *Ciba Found. Symp.* **150,** 112–127 (1990).
64. P. W. Majerus, T. S. Ross, T. W. Cunningham, K. K. Caldwell, A. B. Jefferson, and V. S. Bansal, *Cell* **63,** 459–465 (1990).
65. Y. Emori, Y. Homma, H. Sorimachi, H. Kawasaki, O. Nakanishi, K. Suzuki, and T. Takenawa, *J. Biol. Chem.* **264,** 21885–21890 (1989).
66. S. Ohta, A. Matsui, Y. Nozawa, and Y. Kagawa, *FEBS Lett.* **242,** 31–35 (1988).
67. M. L. Stahl, C. R. Ferenz, K. L. Kelleher, R. W. Kriz, and J. L. Knopf, *Nature (London)* **332,**269–272 (1988).
68. B. J. Mayer, M. Hamaguchi, and H. Hanafusa, *Nature (London)* **332,** 272–275 (1989).
69. S. Nishibe, M. I. Wahl, S. M. T. Hernandez-Sotomayor, N. K. Tonks, S. G. Rhee, and G. Carpenter, *Science* **250,** 1253–1256 (1990).
70. D. A. Kumjian, M. I. Wahl, S. G. Rhee, and T. O. Daniel, *Proc. Natl. Acad. Sci. U.S.A.* **86,** 8232–8236 (1989).
71. B. Margolis, S. G. Rhee, S. Felder, M. Mervic, R. Lyall, A. Levitzki, A. Ullrich, A. Zilberstein, and J. Schlessinger, *Cell* **57,** 1101–1107 (1989).
72. D. K. Morrison, D. R. Kaplan, S. G. Rhee, and L. T. Williams, *Mol. Cell. Biol.* **10,** 2359–2366 (1990).
73. J. Meisenhelder, P.-G. Suh, S. G. Rhee, and T. Hunter, *Cell* **57,** 1109–1122 (1989).
74. B. Margolis, A. Zilberstein, C. Franks, S. Felder, S. Dremer, A. Ullrich, S. G. Rhee, K. Skorecki, and J. Schlessinger, *Science* **248,** 607–610 (1990).
75. M. R. Smith, S.-H. Ryu, P.-G. Suh, S. G. Rhee, and H.-F. Kung, *Proc. Natl. Acad. Sci. U.S.A.* **86,** 3659–3663 (1989).
76. M. R. Smith, Y.-L. Liu, H. Kim, S. G. Rhee, and H.-F. Kung, *Science* **247,** 1074–1077 (1990).
77. B. T. Bloomquist, R. D. Shortridge, S. Schneuwly, M. Perdew, C. Montell, H. Steller, G. Rubin, and W. L. Pak, *Cell* **54,** 723–733 (1988).
78. D. B. Wilson, T. M. Connolly, T.E. Bross, P. W. Majerus, W. R. Sherman, A. N. Tyler, L. J. Rubin, and J. E. Brown, *J. Biol. Chem.* **260,** 13496–13501 (1985).
79. B. J. Stith and W. R. Proctor, *J. Cell. Biochem.* **40,** 321–330 (1989).
80. R. F. Irvine, A. J. Letcher, D. J. Lander, and M. J. Berridge, *Biochem. J.* **240,** 917–920 (1986).
81. C. H. Lee and L. E. Hokin, *Biochem. Biophys. Res. Commun.* **159,** 561–565 (1989).
82. A. R. Hughes, H. Takemura, and J. W. Putney, Jr., *J. Biol. Chem.* **263,** 10314–10319 (1988).
83. J. F. Dixon and L. E. Hokin, *J. Biol. Chem.* **264,** 11721–11724 (1989).
84. J. W. Kim, S.-H. Ryu, and S.-G. Rhee, *Biochem. Biophys. Res. Commun.* **163,** 177–182 (1989).
85. T. M. Connolly, V. S. Bansal, T. E. Bross, R. F. Irvine, and P. W. Majerus, *J. Biol. Chem.* **262,** 2146–2149 (1987).
86. V. S. Bansal, K. Caldwell, and P. W. Majerus, *J. Biol. Chem.* **265,** 1806–1811 (1990).
87. T. S. Ross and P. W. Majerus, *J. Biol. Chem.* **261,** 11119–11123 (1986).
88. T. S. Ross, J. F. Tait, and P. W. Majerus, *Science* **248,** 605–607 (1990).
89. T. S. Ross and P. W. Majerus, *J. Biol. Chem.* **266,** 851–866 (1991).
90. J. Glenny, *J. Biol. Chem.* **261,** 7247–7252 (1986).
91. W. R. Sherman, *in* "Inositol Lipids in Cell Signaling" (R. H. Michell, A. H. Drummond, and C. P. Downes, eds.), pp. 39–79. Academic Press, San Diego, California, 1989.
92. T. S. Ross, B. Whiteley, R. A. Graham, and P. W. Majerus, *J. Biol. Chem.* **266,** 9086–9092 (1991).
93. R. F. Irvine, A. J. Letcher, D. J. Lander, and C. P. Downes, *Biochem. J.* **223,** 237–243 (1984).
94. R. F. Irvine, E. E. Anggard, A. J. Letcher, and C. P. Downes, *Biochem. J.* **229,** 505–511 (1985).

95. G. M. Burgess, J. S. McKinney, R. F. Irvine, and J. W. Putney, Jr., *Biochem. J.* **232,** 237–243 (1985).
96. I. R. Batty, S. R. Nahorski, and R. F. Irvine, *Biochem. J.* **232,** 211–215 (1985).
97. C. A. Hansen, S. Mah, and J. R. Williamson, *J. Biol. Chem.* **261,** 8100–8103 (1986).
98. S. J. Stewart, V. Prpic, F. S. Powers, S. B. Bocckino, R. E. Isaacks, and J. H. Exton, *Proc. Natl. Acad. Sci. U.S.A.* **83,** 6098–6102 (1986).
99. K. A. Tennes, J. S. McKinney, and J. W. Putney, Jr., *Biochem. J.* **242,** 797–802 (1987).
100. R. F. Irvine, A. J. Letcher, J. P. Heslop, and M. J. Berridge, *Nature (London)* **320,** 631–634 (1986).
101. A. B. Theibert, S. Supattapone, C. D. Ferris, S. K. Danoff, R. K. Evans, and S. H. Snyder, *Biochem. J.* **267,** 441–445 (1990).
102. A. P. Morris, D. V. Gallacher, R. F. Irvine, and O. H. Peterson, *Nature (London)* **330,**653–655 (1987).
103. R. F. Irvine and R. M. Moor, *Biochem. J.* **240,** 917–920 (1986).
104. K. H. Moon, S. Y. Lee, and S. G. Rhee, *Biochem. Biophys. Res. Commun.* **163,** 177–182 (1989).
105. T. J. Biden, B. Peter-Riesch, W. Schlegel, and C. B. Wollheim, *J. Biol. Chem.* **262,** 3567–3571 (1987).
106. K. Yamaguchi, M. Hirata, and H. Kuriyama, *Biochem. J.* **244,** 787–791 (1987).
107. Y. Kimura, M. Hirata, K. Yamaguchi, and T. Koga, *Arch. Biochem. Biophys.* **257,** 363–369 (1987).
108. A. J. Morris, C. P. Downes, T. K. Harden, and R. H. Michell, *Biochem. J.* **248,** 489–493 (1987).
109. S.-H. Ryu, S. Y. Lee, K. Y. Lee, and S. G. Rhee, *FASEB J.* **1,** 388–393.
110. R. M. Johnson, W. J. Wasilenko, R. R. Mattingly, M. J. Weber, and J. C. Garrison, *Science* **246,** 121–124 (1989).
111. K. Y. Choi, H. K. Kim, S. Y. Lee, K. H. Moon, S. S. Sim, J. W. Kim, H. K. Chung, and S. G. Rhee, *Science* **248,** 64–66 (1990).
112. T. J. Biden, J. G. Altin, A. Karajalainen, and F. L. Bygrave, *Biochem. J.* **256,** 697–701 (1988).
113. L. M. Molina y Vedia and E. G. Lapetina, *J. Biol. Chem.* **261,** 10493–10495 (1986).
114. T. M. Connolly, T. E. Bross, and P. W. Majerus, *J. Biol. Chem.* **260,** 7868–7874 (1985).
115. C. A. Mitchell, T. M. Connolly, and P. W. Majerus, *J. Biol. Chem.* **264,** 8873–8877 (1989).
116. C. A. Hansen, R. A. Johanson, M. T. Williamson, and J. R. Williamson, *J. Biol. Chem.* **262,** 12319–12326 (1987).
117. K. Takimoto, M. Okada, and H. Nakagawa, *J. Biochem. (Tokyo)* **106,** 684–690 (1989).
118. C. Erneux, M. Lemos, B. Verjans, P. Vanderhaeghen, A. Delvaux, and J. E. Dumont, *Eur. J. Biochem.* **181,** 317–322 (1989).
119. T. S. Ross, C. A. Mitchell, A. B. Jefferson, and P. W. Majerus, *J. Biol. Chem.* **266,** 20283–20289 (1991).
120. S. B. Shears, *Biochem. J.* **260,** 313–324 (1989).
121. T. M. Connolly, W. J. Lawing, and P. W. Majerus, *Cell* **46,** 951–958 (1986).
122. R. C. Inhorn, V. S. Bansal, and P. W. Majerus, *Proc. Natl. Acad. Sci. U.S.A.* **84,** 2170–2174 (1987).
123. V. Sylvia, G. Curtin, J. Norman, J. Stec, and D. Busbee, *Cell* **54,** 651–658 (1988).
124. R. C. Inhorn and P. W. Majerus, *J. Biol. Chem.* **262,** 15946–15952 (1987).
125. N. S. Gee, G. G. Reid, R. G. Jackson, R. J. Barnaby, and C. I. Ragan, *Biochem. J.* **253,** 777–782 (1988).
126. J. D. York and P. W. Majerus, *Proc. Natl. Acad. Sci. U.S.A.* **87,** 9548–9552 (1990).
127. R. C. Inhorn and P. W. Majerus, *J. Biol. Chem.* **263,** 14559–14565 (1988).
128. V. S. Bansal, R. C. Inhorn, and P. W. Majerus, *J. Biol. Chem.* **262,** 9444–9447 (1987).

129. deleted in proof
130. T. Balla, G. Guillemette, A. J. Baukal, and K. J. Catt, *J. Biol. Chem.* **242,** 9952–9955 (1987).
131. L. R. Stephens, P. T. Hawkins, C. J. Barker, and C. P. Downes, *Biochem. J.* **253,** 721–723 (1988).
132. C. A. Hansen, S. V. Dahl, B. Huddell, and J. R. Williamson, *FEBS Lett.* **236,** 53–56 (1988).
133. S. B. Shears, *J. Biol. Chem.* **264,** 19897–19886 (1989).
134. R. E. Diehl, P. Whiting, J. Potter, N. Gee, C. I. Ragan, D. Linemeyer, R. Schoepfer, C. Bennett, and R. A. F. Dixon, *J. Biol. Chem.* **265,** 5946–5949 (1990).
135. K. E. Ackermann, B. G. Gish, M. P. Honchar, and W. R. Sherman, *Biochem. J.* **242,** 517–524 (1987).
136. L. M. Hallcher and W. R. Sherman, *J. Biol. Chem.* **255,** 10896–10901 (1980).
137. R. G. Jackson, N. S. Gee, and C. I. Ragan, *Biochem. J.* **264,** 419–422 (1989).
138. M. J. Berridge, C. P. Downes, and M. R. Hanley, *Cell* **59,** 411–419 (1989).

CHAPTER 7

Phosphatidylinositol 3-kinase: A Novel Signal Transduction Pathway?

Kurt R. Auger and Lewis C. Cantley

Department of Physiology
Tufts University School of Medicine
Boston, Massachusetts 02111

Introduction

Polyphosphoinositides have been extensively studied because of their involvement in intracellular signaling. Phosphatidylinositol 4,5-bisphosphate (PtdIns-4,5-P_2) and phosphatidylinositol 4-phosphate (PtdIns-4-P) are precursors of the second messenger pathway involving inositol 1,4,5-trisphosphate (Ins-1,4,5-P_3) and diacylglycerol (DAG). Recently, a group of polyphosphoinositides containing a phosphate at the D-3 position of the inositol ring has been found. The enzyme primarily responsible for producing these lipids, phosphatidylinositol 3-kinase (PtdIns 3-kinase), was discovered because of a tight physical association with various oncogene products and growth factor receptors with intrinsic protein tyrosine kinase activity. The lipid products of this enzyme are not in the conventional phosphatidylinositol (PtdIns) turnover pathway, but appear to act in a new signaling pathway.

Cellular and Molecular Mechanisms of Inflammation, Volume 3

This review discusses the enzymology and mechanism of regulation of PtdIns 3-kinase, which has been implicated in the control of cell growth and transformation. Phosphoinositide kinases are summarized in more detail in a recent review (Carpenter and Cantley, 1990).

Pathway and Structures for the Conventional Polyphosphoinositides

A large number of extracellular ligands are involved in the regulated breakdown of polyphosphoinositides. Two very well-characterized second messengers are produced as a consequence of ligand–receptor interaction: DAG and Ins-1,4,5-P_3. The production of these two second messengers results from the cleavage of PtdIns-4,5-P_2 by a PtdIns-specific phospholipase C (PtdIns-PLC). DAG activates the Ca^{2+}/phospholipid-dependent serine/threonine protein kinase C (PKC), and Ins-1,4,5-P_3 releases Ca^{2+} from intracellular stores. PtdIns-4,5-P_2 is formed from the sequential phosphorylation of PtdIns and then PtdIns-4-P by phosphatidylinositol 4-kinase (PtdIns 4-kinase) and PtdIns-4-P 5-kinase, respectively (see Fig. 1).

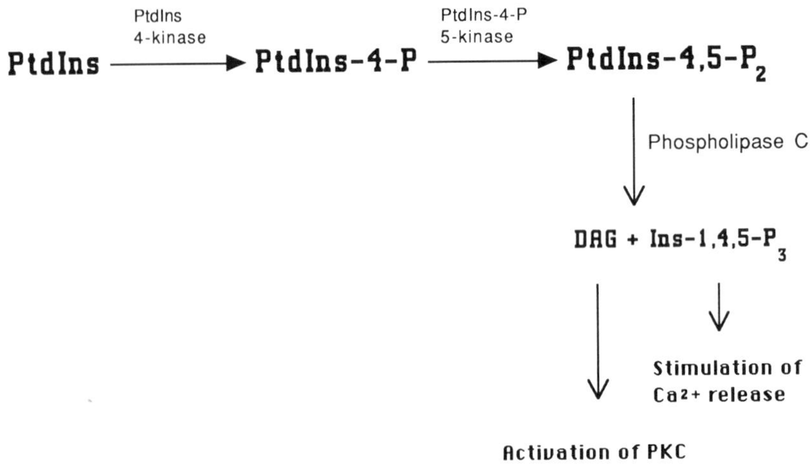

FIGURE 1

The conventional phosphoinositide pathway. PtdIns-4,5-P_2 is formed by sequential phosphorylation of PtdIns and is a substrate for phospholipase C. The hydrolysis products, diacylglycerol (DAG) and Ins-1,4,5-P_3, activate protein kinase C (PKC) and stimulate Ca^{2+} release, respectively.

Since the early reports of mitogenic stimulation of lymphocytes by Fisher and Mueller (1968) and of retroviral transformation by Diringer and Friis (1977), many studies have linked stimulated phosphoinositide turnover with cellular proliferation. The relationship between cell proliferation and general phosphoinositide metabolism has been extensively reviewed (see, e.g., Berridge, 1987; Rana and Hokin, 1990; Weinstein, 1987; Whitman and Cantley, 1988).

PtdIns is 1,2-diacyl-*sn*-3-glycerophosphoryl D-1 *myo*-inositol; in mammalian cells the acyl chains are often stearoyl (C_{18}) at the 1 position and arachidonoyl (C_{20}; 5,8,11,14) at the 2 position of glycerol. Figure 2A shows the structure of PtdIns. PtdIns-4-P and PtdIns-4,5-P_2 are the products of sequential phosphorylation of PtdIns and PtdIns-4-P by distinct enzymes (see Fig. 1). The structures of these polyphosphoinositides are shown in Fig. 2B and C.

A Distinct Phosphatidylinositol Kinase Associates with Activated Protein Tyrosine Kinases

The initial report that showed evidence of a direct association between a protein tyrosine kinase and PtdIns kinase activity was provided by Sugimoto *et al.* (1984). A highly purified preparation of pp60$^{v\text{-}src}$ had PtdIns, PtdInsP, and DAG kinase activities that could be inhibited in parallel with inhibition of the protein tyrosine kinase activity. In addition, previous work had shown that similar preparations of pp60$^{v\text{-}src}$ had the ability to phosphorylate low-molecular-weight alcohols, including glycerol (Graziani *et al.*, 1983; Richert *et al.*, 1982). These early results led to the suggestion that pp60$^{v\text{-}src}$ itself was responsible for the lipid kinase activity. However, subsequent work established that pp60$^{v\text{-}src}$ expressed *in vitro* lacked the lipid kinase activity and that a tightly associated protein(s) from the host cell was responsible for the lipid kinase activity (Kaplan *et al.*, 1987; Piwnica-Worms *et al.*, 1986).

Concurrent work by Macara *et al.* (1984) demonstrated that PtdIns kinase activity immunoprecipitated with p68$^{v\text{-}ros}$, the transforming protein of the avian sarcoma virus UR2. This protein, like pp60$^{v\text{-}src}$, is a protein tyrosine kinase.

Whitman *et al.* (1985) demonstrated that the middle T antigen (mT) of polyoma virus that associated with and activated the cellular homolog of pp60$^{v\text{-}src}$ (pp60$^{c\text{-}src}$) also associated with an active PtdIns kinase. The PtdIns kinase activity could be immunoprecipitated from transformed cells, but

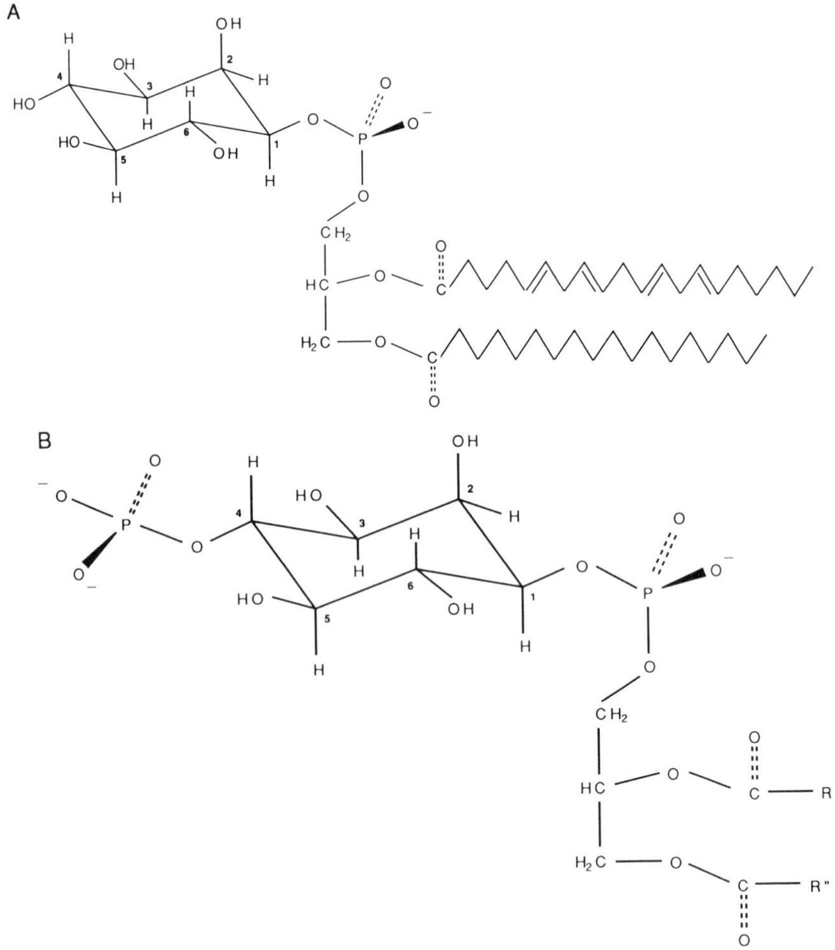

FIGURE 2

Structure of the various polyphosphoinositides. (A) Structure of phosphatidylinositol (1,2-diacyl-*sn*-3-glycerophosphoryl D-1 *myo*-inositol. Also shown are structures of (B) phosphatidylinositol 4-phosphate, (C) phosphatidylinositol 4,5-bisphosphate, (D) phosphatidylinositol 3-phosphate, (E) phosphatidylinositol 3,4-bisphosphate, and (F) phosphatidylinositol 3,4,5-trisphosphate. R and R″ represent the fatty acyl chains found in phosphatidylinositol: R″, Stearoyl; R, arachidonoyl.

C

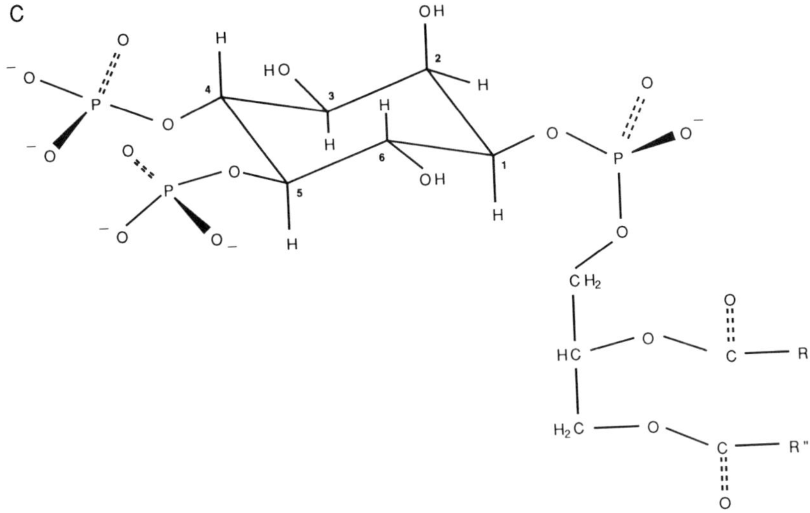

D

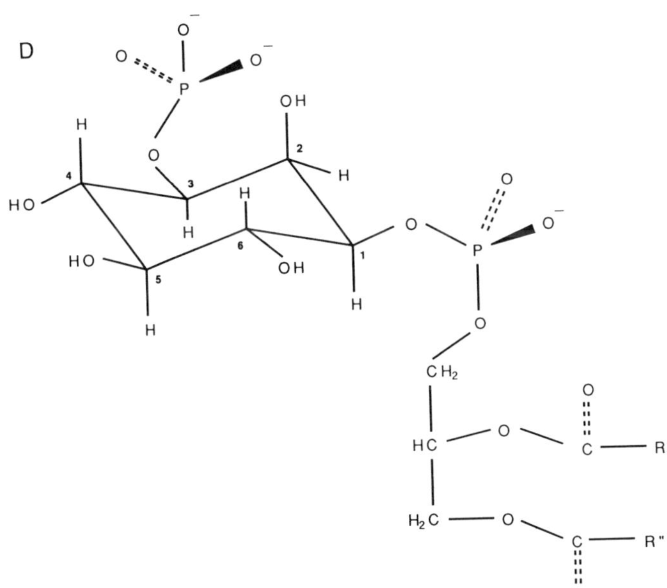

FIGURE 2

continued

E

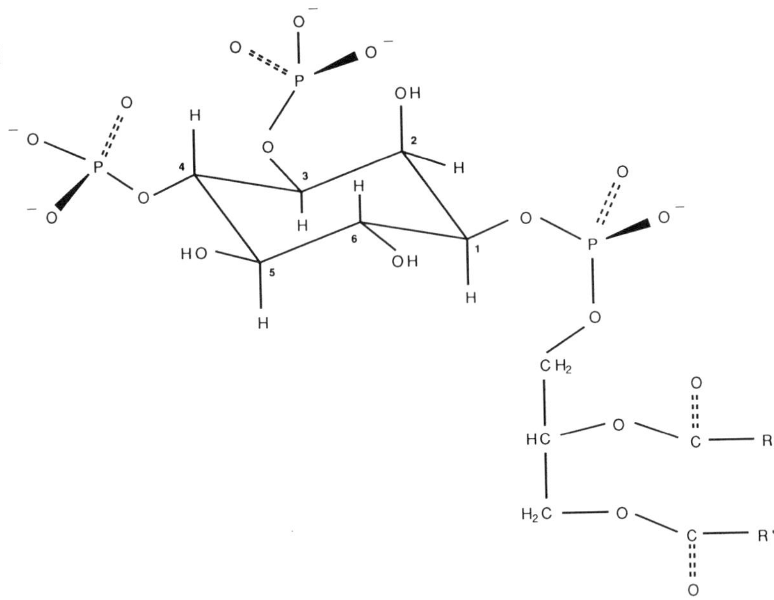

F

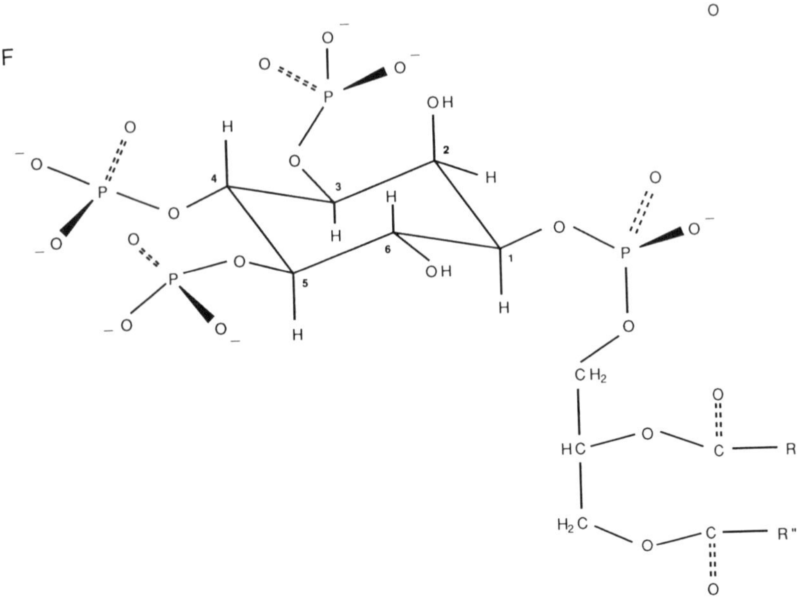

FIGURE 2 *continued*

not from mock-infected controls (Whitman *et al.*, 1985), using either anti-mT antiserum or anti-pp60^{src} monoclonal antibodies.

PtdIns kinase activity was also detected in v-*abl* protein tyrosine kinase immunoprecipitates from Abelson-transformed cells (Fry *et al.*, 1985). Thus, a correlation between the association of PtdIns kinase activity and protein tyrosine kinases involved in cell transformation was established.

A further characterization of PtdIns kinases in fibroblasts revealed the existence of two distinct enzymes, only one of which associated with protein tyrosine kinases. The two PtdIns kinase activities from whole-cell lysates could be separated by a Mono Q (Pharmacia, Piscataway, NJ) anion-exchange fast protein liquid chromatography column. The two enzymatic activities differed with respect to inhibition by adenosine, K_m for ATP, and sensitivity to nonionic detergents (Whitman *et al.*, 1987). The activities could also be differentiated by their ability to associate specifically with the activated protein tyrosine kinases pp60$^{v\text{-}src}$ and mT/pp60$^{c\text{-}src}$. The PtdIns kinase activity which eluted first from the Mono Q column (designated type I) was the activity that associated with protein tyrosine kinases and was inhibited by detergent. The PtdIns kinase activity which eluted from the anion-exchange column at higher salt concentration (designated type II) was inhibited by adenosine and was activated by nonionic detergents (Whitman *et al.*, 1987). In addition, the type II PtdIns kinase activity bound non specifically to Sepharose (Sigma Chemical Corp., St. Louis, MO) beads commonly used in immunoprecipitations (Jackowski *et al.*, 1986; Whitman *et al.*, 1987) and could be removed by washing with NP-40 (Sigma Chemical Corp., St. Louis, MO) (Whitman *et al.*, 1987). The type II PtdIns kinase activity was the more abundant activity in the cell.

Type I PtdIns kinase activity was also linked to tyrosine-phosphorylated proteins in nontransformed cells with the observation that this activity copurified with the activated platelet-derived growth factor (PDGF) receptor in PDGF-stimulated cells. Wheat germ lectin- and antiphosphotyrosine (α-P-tyr)-purified PDGF receptor from stimulated fibroblasts contained type I PtdIns kinase activity (Whitman *et al.*, 1987). However, the activity was not present in the partially purified preparations if the cells were not stimulated with PDGF prior to purification.

An exciting breakthrough came with the finding that type I PtdIns kinase phosphorylated PtdIns to produce a previously undescribed PtdInsP, PtdIns-3-P, instead of the conventional PtdIns-4-P product (Whitman *et al.*, 1988). Initially, the novel product appeared to comigrate with PtdIns-4-P on both one- and two-dimensional thin-layer chromatography systems. More careful analysis revealed that the PtdInsP produced by the type I enzyme migrated slightly more slowly than the PtdInsP produced by the type II PtdIns kinase using the standard chloroform:methanol:ammonium hydroxide thin-layer chromatography solvent system (Whitman *et al.*, 1988). The fatty acyl side chains of the two products were examined by reversed-phase high-performance liquid chromatography (HPLC) and were found to have similar distributions. A difference was found when the inositol head group of the two products was examined to determine the location of the incorporated phosphate. Deacylation of the novel PtdInsP to remove the fatty acyl chains produced a glycerophosphoinositol phosphate (gPtdInsP) that had a distinctly different retention time on strong anion-exchange HPLC from that of the gPtdInsP produced from deacylating PtdIns-4-P. In addition, when deacylation of the novel gPtdInsP was followed by mild periodate treatment (deglyceration), the inositol bisphosphate ($InsP_2$) that resulted was distinct from the product of deacylated and deglycerated PtdIns-4-P (Whitman *et al.*, 1988). The different retention times on the strong anion-exchange HPLC column provided evidence that the type I PtdIns kinase phosphorylated a different position of the inositol ring than the conventional PtdIns kinase typically found in cells.

The $InsP_2$ produced after deacylating and deglycerating the products of the type I and type II PtdIns kinases was incubated with 100 m*M* sodium periodate, reduced with borohydride, and then treated with phosphatase to generate polyols that could be identified by HPLC on a Brownlee polybore carbohydrate column by comigration with standards. The polyol produced from the novel PtdInsP could only result if the starting lipid was phosphorylated at the D-1 and D-3 positions of *myo*-inositol. Thus, the starting material was PtdIns-3-P (Whitman *et al.*, 1988). The structure of PtdIns-3-P is shown in Fig. 2D.

The generation of PtdIns-3-P as discussed above was from *in vitro* immunoprecipitates. Whitman *et al.* (1988) also showed that an inositol lipid with properties identical to those of PtdIns-3-P was present in intact fibroblasts. Cells transformed with mT were labeled with [^{3}H]inositol and the phospholipids were extracted and deacylated for subsequent HPLC analysis. A peak that comigrated with [^{32}P]gPtdIns-3-P generated *in vitro* was detected and constituted 3.3% of the total PtdInsP in the [^{3}H]inositol-labeled cells (Whitman *et al.*, 1988). The structure of PtdIns-3-P extracted from *in vivo* labeled cells was confirmed by analysis of lipids from astrocytoma cells (Stephens *et al.*, 1989). Stephens *et al.* (1989) also found that the turnover rate of PtdIns-3-P was similar to the rate of turnover for the conventional polyphosphoinositides. This suggested that PtdIns-3-P, PtdIns-4-P, and PtdIns-4,5-P_2 were synthesized from a common pool of phosphatidyl-*myo*-inositol (Stephens *et al.*, 1989).

The discoveries that a novel PtdInsP was produced by type I PtdIns kinase and that this kinase was directly associated with protein tyrosine kinases such as growth factor receptors and activated oncogene products led to the proposal that PtdIns-3-P, or a metabolite, could be a mitogenic signal for these protein tyrosine kinases.

Phosphatidylinositol 3-kinase Is Linked to Cell Proliferation and Transformation

The previous discussion illustrates the association of a PtdIns kinase activity with the activated protein tyrosine kinases $pp60^{v\text{-}src}$ (Kaplan *et al.*, 1986; Sugimoto *et al.*, 1984), $pp68^{v\text{-}ros}$ (Macara *et al.*, 1984), and v-*abl* (Fry *et al.*, 1985) and the mT/$pp60^{c\text{-}src}$ complex (Kaplan *et al.*, 1986; Whitman *et al.*, 1985). Examination of various polyoma mT mutants provided convincing evidence that PtdIns 3-kinase was important for cell transformation.

The nontransforming mT mutants NG59 and py1387T do not have associated PtdIns kinase activity and also do not activate $pp60^{c\text{-}src}$ (Kaplan *et al.*, 1986; Whitman *et al.*, 1985). Polyoma mutant py1178T is characterized as having a host range-specific defect in transformation; however, py1178T is still capable of associating with and activating $pp60^{c\text{-}src}$ (Carmichael *et al.*, 1984; Oostra *et al.*, 1983). When this mutant was examined for PtdIns kinase activity, an intermediate level of kinase activity was detected (Whitman *et al.*, 1985). Three other important mutants—dl23, dl1015, and dl1014/py1178T—were found to associate with and activate $pp60^{c\text{-}src}$ to wild-type levels of protein tyrosine kinase activity, but they were only partially transformation competent. These mutants had intermediate levels of PtdIns kinase activity compared with transformation-competent wild-type mT, much like the previously described py1178T mutant (Whitman *et al.*, 1985). $pp60^{c\text{-}src}$ immunoprecipitates from cells transformed with simian virus 40 large T antigen or an activated c-*ras* gene did not have increased PtdIns kinase activity. Thus, these results provide evidence that the association of $pp60^{c\text{-}src}$ and PtdIns kinase was not a general phenomenon of the transformed phenotype, but instead was specific to mT or v-*src* transformation (Kaplan *et al.*, 1986).

Mutational studies with the PDGF receptor suggest that PtdIns 3-kinase is functionally important for regulated cell proliferation. The PDGF receptor is the prototype for a family of protein tyrosine kinase growth factor receptors. This receptor family has a "kinase insert" region which divides the conserved kinase domain (Williams, 1989). Removal of the kinase insert region and transfection of this mutant receptor (ΔKI) into Chinese hamster ovary cells illustrates the importance of PtdIns 3-kinase to cell proliferation. Cells transfected with either the wild-type of ΔKI receptor and stimulated with PDGF had similar responses with respect to PDGF binding, protein tyrosine kinase activity, pH change, accumulation of inositol phosphates, and Ca^{2+} mobilization. However, PDGF did not stimulate incorporation of [^{3}H]thymidine and cause an increase in cell number in cells transfected with the ΔKI mutants (Escobedo and Williams, 1988). It was later shown that the ΔKI mutant could not associate with PtdIns 3-kinase (Coughlin *et al.*, 1989).

Since PtdIns kinase was found to be associated with activated protein tyrosine kinases, but not with nontransforming mT mutants, the ΔKI mutant, or the unstimulated PDGF receptor, it was possible to find a candidate polypeptide for type I PtdIns kinase. Kaplan *et al.* (1987) suggested that an 85-kDa phosphoprotein, common to mT/pp60$^{c\text{-}src}$ and PDGF receptor immunoprecipitates, was the putative PtdIns kinase or one of its subunits. Indeed, the 85-kDa polypeptides detected in both types of immunoprecipitates were shown to be very similar or identical by V8 and chymotrypsin protease mapping. The 85-kDa polypeptide was also shown to be phosphorylated both *in vitro* in immune complex kinase reactions and *in vivo* by $^{32}P_i$ labeling. Both labeling procedures produced labeled phosphoserine and phosphotyrosine residues. Neither the 85-kDa protein nor PtdIns kinase activity could be detected in α-P-tyr immunoprecipitates from epidermal growth factor (EGF)-stimulated or simian virus 40 T antigen-transformed cells. However, both the polypeptide and PtdIns kinase activity were detected in α-P-tyr immunoprecipitates from cells transformed with v-*fms* and v-*sis* (Kaplan *et al.*, 1987).

Courtneidge and Heber (1987) also observed a correlation between the appearance of PtdIns kinase activity and an 81-kDa polypeptide in mT/pp60$^{c\text{-}src}$ immunoprecipitates from cells containing various mT mutants. p81 was shown to be phosphorylated exclusively on tyrosine residues in the immune complex protein kinase reaction and was also found in immunoprecipitates from $^{32}P_i$-labeled cells. The presence of this protein and the correlation with PtdIns kinase activity in a number of mT mutants suggested that p81 was the PtdIns kinase (Courtneidge and Heber, 1987).

The association of PtdIns 3-kinase activity with activated protein tyrosine kinases correlated with the mitogenic response. However, the mere association of PtdIns 3-kinase activity with an activity protein tyrosine kinase was soon shown to be insufficient for mitogenesis. Although the association of PtdIns kinase activity with pp60$^{v\text{-}src}$ had been reported as early as 1984 (Sugimoto *et al.*, 1984), the formal identification that the product of the lipid kinase assay was PtdIns-3-P was not confirmed until later by Fukui and Hanafusa (1989). More importantly, a myristylation-defective mutant, although still associated with PtdIns 3-kinase, was defective in transformation (Fukui and Hanafusa, 1989).

A second example that association of PtdIns 3-kinase with an activated protein tyrosine kinase was insufficient for mitogenesis was based on the observation that the colony-stimulating factor 1 (CSF-1) receptor associates with PtdIns 3-kinase (Varticovski *et al.*, 1989). Mutation of Tyr-809 to phenylalanine in the human CSF-1 receptor resulted in the inability to transduce a mitogenic signal, even though the receptor was active as a protein tyrosine kinase, associated with PtdIns 3-kinase activity, and induced the expression of the protooncogenes c-*fos* and *junB* (Roussel *et al.*, 1990).

The final example which showed that association of PtdIns 3-kinase with an activated protein tyrosine kinase is not sufficient for transformation was provided by a previously undescribed polyoma mT mutant. This mutant was characterized as having a single amino acid substitution: Pro-248 was converted to leucine (Druker *et al.*, 1990). This mT mutant not only activated the protein tyrosine kinase activity of $pp60^{c\text{-}src}$ to wild-type levels, but also associated with PtdIns 3-kinase. In addition, the *in vitro* PtdIns 3-kinase activity was similar to the kinase activity in immunoprecipitates of wild type mT (Druker *et al.*, 1990). Thus, it appears, from mutational studies of various protein tyrosine kinases, that association of PtdIns 3-kinase with protein tyrosine kinases is necessary, but not sufficient for mitogenesis.

The importance of PtdIns 3-kinase to fundamental cellular metabolism was investigated by determining the evolutionary conservation of this enzymatic activity. Evidence has been found that PtdIns 3-kinase activity is conserved in the budding yeast *Saccharomyces cerevisiae* (Auger *et al.*, 1989a). *In vitro* PtdIns kinase assays of yeast cell homogenates with subsequent HPLC analysis of the deacylated lipid showed the presence of PtdIns 3-kinase activity. Preliminary biochemical characterization of the activity demonstrated that the yeast enzyme differed from the mammalian enzyme, yet the phosphorylation of PtdIns at the D-3 position of the inositol ring was conserved. *In vivo* [^{3}H]inositol labeling of intact *S. cerevisiae* demonstrated that PtdIns-3-P was as abundant as PtdIns-4-P in the yeast cell membranes (Auger *et al.*, 1989a). Thus, PtdIns 3-kinase appears to play an important role in species as diverse as yeast and mammals.

Discovery of Other Novel Polyphosphoinositides

The finding of PtdIns 3-kinase and its novel product, PtdIns-3-P, in intact cells led to questions about its metabolism (Stephens *et al.*, 1989; Whitman *et al.*, 1988). Previous studies had failed to find polyphosphoinositides other than PtdIns-4-P and PtdIns-4,5-P_2 (Downes *et al.*, 1986; Hawkins *et al.*, 1986).

In addition to PtdIns-3-P two other novel polyphosphoinositides could be produced by activities in α-P-tyr immunoprecipitates from PDGF-stimulated cells (Auger *et al.*, 1989b). The same phospholipids were also produced *in vivo* when smooth muscle cells were stimulated with PDGF. These polyphosphoinositides were tentatively identified as phosphatidylinositol 3,4-bisphosphate (PtdIns-3,4-P_2) and phosphatidylinositol 3,4,5-trisphosphate (PtdIns-3,4,5-P_3) based on comigration of the deacylated and deglycerated compounds with [^{3}H]inositol standards on strong anion-exchange HPLC. It was also suggested that a single enzyme, PtdIns 3-kinase, in the α-P-tyr immunoprecipitate produced these polyphosphoinositides by using PtdIns, PtdIns-4-P, and PtdIns-4,5-P_2 as substrates, respectively. This hypothesis has been substantiated, as PtdIns 3-kinase purified to homogeneity can utilize all three lipids as substrates (Carpenter *et al.*, 1990). The structures of PtdIns-3,4-P_2 and PtdIns-3,4,5-P_3 produced by the purified PtdIns 3-kinase have been confirmed by phosphatase treatment of the deacylated and deglycerated products (Auger, 1991). Structures of PtdIns-3,4-P_2 and PtdIns-3,4,5-P_3 produced *in vivo* by platelets were also confirmed (Cunningham *et al.*, 1990). Figure 2E and F depicts the structures of PtdIns-3,4-P_2 and PtdIns-3,4,5-P_3. The hypothesis that the 85-kDa phosphoprotein common to the PDGF receptor and mT immunoprecipitates is a subunit of the PtdIns 3-kinase was also verified. Purified PtdIns 3-kinase was shown to be a heterodimer of the previously discussed 85-kDa protein and a 110-kDa protein (Carpenter *et al.*, 1990).

Elevation of the novel polyphosphoinositides also occurred as a result of transformation of fibroblasts by polyoma mT (Serunian *et al.*, 1990; Ulug *et al.*, 1990). The appearance of PtdIns-3,4-P_2 and PtdIns-3,4,5-P_3 was dependent on the expression of protein tyrosine kinase activity associated with mT, as demonstrated by the induction of mT on a dexamethasone expression vector (Serunian *et al.*, 1990). PtdIns-3,4-P_2 and PtdIns-3,4,5-P_3were present in transformed cells at high density, but were not detected in nontransformed parent cells at high density and subject to density-dependent growth arrest. Thus, the presence of these novel polyphosphoinositides correlates with cell proliferation as a result of either mitogenic stimulation or transformation.

The metabolic fate of the D-3 phosphorylated polyphosphoinositides is currently unknown. However, it has been shown that the various phospholipase C (PLC) enzymes that have been purified and/or cloned do not utilize these polyphosphoinositides as substrates (Lips *et al.*, 1989; Serunian *et al.*, 1989). It should be noted that a 3-phosphomonoesterate that hydrolyzes PtdIns-3-P has been reported (Lips and Majerus, 1989).

A number of studies have found compounds with HPLC chromatographic properties similar to those of PtdIns-3,4-P_2 and PtdIns-3,4,5-P_3. Stimulated neutrophils appear to have PtdIns-3,4-P_2 and PtdIns-3,4,5-P_3(Traynor-Kaplan *et al.*, 1988, 1989). Evidence for PtdIns-3,4-P_2 in MA-10 Leydig tumor cells has been found in response to stimulation by EGF (Pignataro and Ascoli, 1990). In addition, three other groups described compounds similar to PtdIns-3,4-P_2 and PtdIns-3,4,5-P_3 in stimulated platelets (Cunningham *et al.*, 1990; Kucera and Rittenhouse, 1990; Nolan and Lapetina, 1990, 1991). An early indication that PtdInsP_3 was found in $^{32}P_i$ labeled brain (Santiago-Calvo *et al.*, 1963) was not confirmed after further investigation (Santiago-Calvo *et al.*, 1964). However, recent evidence suggests that PtdInsP_3 is present in brain tissue (Vadnal and Parthasarathy, 1989).

An enzymatic activity that converts PtdIns-3-P to PtdIns-3,4-P_2 was recently discovered in platelets (Yamamoto *et al.*, 1990) and red blood cells (Graziani *et al.*, 1992). The PtdIns-3,4-P_2 produced in response to thrombin stimulation of platelets is due to this enzyme (Cunningham *et al.*, 1990). In contrast, PDGF probably induces PtdIns-3,4-P_2 and PtdIns-3,4,5-P_3 production by stimulating phosphorylation of the D-3 position of PtdIns-4-P and PtdIns-4,5-P_2 (Fig. 3). Thus, at least two pathways exist for making these lipids.

Critical Determinants for Association of Phosphatidylinositol 3-kinase and Protein Tyrosine Kinases

As previously discussed, PtdIns 3-kinase activity specifically associates with pp60$^{v\text{-}src}$, p68$^{v\text{-}ros}$, mT/pp60$^{c\text{-}src}$, the stimulated PDGF receptor, and the CSF-1 receptor. Association with the stimulated insulin receptor, p130$^{gag\text{-}fps}$, p47$^{gag\text{-}crk}$, and the mT/pp62$^{c\text{-}yes}$ have also been reported (Fukui *et al.*, 1989; Ruderman *et al.*, 1990). The stimulated EGF receptor also associates with PtdIns 3-kinase in some cell types (Bjorge *et al.*, 1990; Pignataro and Ascoli, 1990), but not others (Kaplan *et al.*, 1987) (L. C. Cantley, unpublished observations). The reason for cell type-specific associations is unclear, but may be related to tissue-specific expression of PtdIns 3-kinase isozymes.

Although PtdIns 3-kinase does not associate with pp60$^{c\text{-}src}$ in nontransformed cells (in which it is relatively inactive as a protein tyrosine kinase), it will associate with pp60$^{c\text{-}src}$ under activating conditions. Association of PtdIns 3-kinase activity with mutationally activated pp60$^{c\text{-}src}$ has been

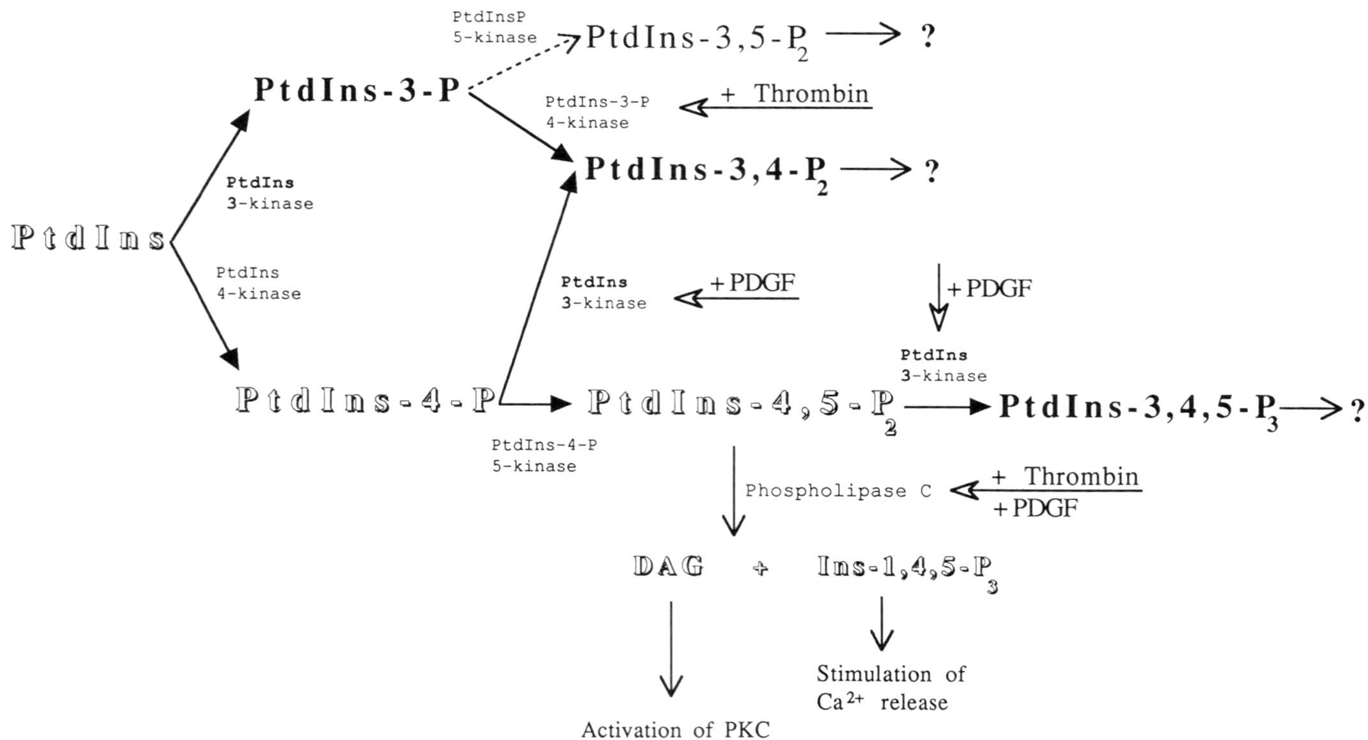

FIGURE 3

Polyphosphoinositide pathways. Schematic diagram of the metabolism of the polyphosphoinositides. Solid arrows indicate the known routes of *in vitro* phosphorylation that produce the indicated polyphosphoinositides. PtdIns-3,5-P_2 is a tentative structural assignment for a lipid that can be produced *in vitro* by phosphorylating PtdIns-3-P with a PtdInsP 5-kinase. Question marks indicate the unknown metabolic fate of the compound. Steps stimulated by platelet-derived growth factor (PDGF) and thrombin are indicated. The conventional pathway is illustrated in outline font. DAG, Diacylglycerol; PKC, protein kinase C.

found (Chan *et al.*, 1990). The association of PtdIns 3-kinase activity was related to the protein tyrosine kinase activity of $pp60^{c\text{-}src}$ rather than to the amount of protein expressed in the cell (Chan *et al.*, 1990). A second and probably more physiological finding was the association of PtdIns 3-kinase activity with $pp60^{c\text{-}src}$ in thrombin-stimulated platelets (Gutkind *et al.*, 1990). PtdIns 3-kinase was also found to associate with another member of the *src* family, $p59^{fyn}$, in a thrombin-dependent manner (Gutkind *et al.*, 1990). The effect was rapid, as PtdIns 3-kinase activity was detected 5 sec after thrombin stimulation.

The interesting observation in all of the above cases is that it appears that an active protein tyrosine kinase is necessary for association of PtdIns 3-kinase activity. We have used immunopurified baculovirus-expressed $mT/pp60^{c\text{-}src}$ complex (Piwnica-Worms *et al.*, 1990) and purified PtdIns 3-kinase (Carpenter *et al.*, 1990) to reconstitute this interaction *in vitro*. Both the 85- and 110-kDa proteins of PtdIns 3-kinase were stoichiometrically associated with the $mT/pp60^{c\text{-}src}$ complex (Auger, 1991). The association was dependent on the active protein tyrosine kinase activity of $pp60^{c\text{-}src}$, as a kinase-deficient mutant, $mT/pp60^{295c\text{-}src}$, did not associate with purified PtdIns 3-kinase. The immunopurified $mT/pp60^{c\text{-}src}$ complex was also found to associate with PtdIns 3-kinase from whole-cell lysates. In addition, the reconstituted PtdIns 3-kinase–$mT/pp60^{c\text{-}src}$ complex produced the same polyphosphoinositides as were produced by kinase activity in α-P-tyr or anti-mT immunoprecipitates from mT-transformed fibroblasts.

The importance of tyrosine phosphorylation on mT has recently been demonstrated for the association of mT with pp85 (Cohen *et al.*, 1990). Tyr-315 of the mT sequence is the major phosphorylation site of mT by $pp60^{c\text{-}src}$; a Tyr→Phe substitution at this site reduces the association of PtdIns 3-kinase activity (Whitman *et al.*, 1985). This mT mutant is transformation defective both *in vitro* (Carmichael *et al.*, 1984; Oostra *et al.*, 1983) and *in vivo* (Talmage *et al.*, 1989). Cohen *et al.* (1990) showed that phosphorylated denatured mT was able to reassociate with pp85 either in solution or by Western blotting after denaturation of cellular proteins. The unphosphorylated form of mT did not reassociate with pp85. Since Tyr-315 of mT in the kinase-defective $mT/pp60^{295c\text{-}src}$ complex is not phosphorylated (Piwnica-Worms *et al.*, 1990), it is likely that this phosphorylation plays a crucial role in the association both *in vitro* (Auger, 1991; Carpenter *et al.*, 1990; Cohen *et al.*, 1990) and *in vivo* (Talmage *et al.*, 1989; Whitman *et al.*, 1985). The contribution of phosphorylation on either c-*src* or the PtdIns 3-kinase complex has yet to be systematically investigated.

The KI region of the PDGF receptor has a short sequence with similarity to the region around Tyr-315 of mT. As discussed previously, this region of the receptor appears to be essential for PtdIns 3-kinase association and mitogenesis (Coughlin *et al.*, 1989). A more detailed investigation revealed that mutating Tyr-751 to phenylalanine or glycine prevented association with PtdIns 3-kinase activity (Kazlauskas and Cooper, 1989). Further characterization of this interaction was investigated by *in vitro* reconstitution. Binding of PtdIns 3-kinase was dependent on phosphorylation of Tyr-751 and was rapid and saturable (Kazlauskas and Cooper, 1990). Based on these studies and a comparison of primary protein sequences of various protein tyrosine kinases known to associate with PtdIns 3-kinase, a consensus sequence (shown in single-letter code) has been implicated to be critical for PtdIns 3-kinase binding: E/D·E/D·E/D·E/D·E/D·$\mathbf{Y}^{PO_4}$·M/V·P·**M**·X·X (Cantley *et al.*, 1991).

Conclusions

This review has discussed the existence of newly described polyphosphoinositides that are responsive to mitogen stimulation or oncogenic transformation in cultured mammalian cells. The time course of production of these novel polyphosphoinositides suggests that they are important signaling molecules in the signal transduction pathway for mitogenic protein tyrosine kinases. The structures of these polyphosphoinositides, PtdIns-3,4-P_2 and PtdIns-3,4,5-P_3, provide evidence that they are not direct precursors for the well-characterized second messenger Ins-1,4,5-P_3. Since the purified PtdIns 3-kinase can utilize PtdIns, PtdIns-4-P, and PtdIns-4,5-P_2 as substrates *in vitro*, it seems likely that activation of PtdIns 3-kinase may result in the generation of multiple signals which branch off from the conventional polyphosphoinositide pathway (Fig. 3), as originally proposed (Auger *et al.*, 1989b). Comparison of Figs. 1 and 3 illustrates the increasing complexity of polyphosphoinositide metabolism. In addition, the observation that the PtdIns 3-kinase pathway also exists in *S. cerevisiae* argues that it plays an important role conserved in eukaryotic cells (Auger *et al.*, 1989a). The exact nature of how these molecules act as messengers has yet to be elucidated; however, some insights are currently being evaluated.

Possible Functions of the Novel Polyphosphoinositides

Currently, no specific function(s) has been assigned to PtdIns-3,4-P_2 and PtdIns-3,4,5-P_3. As discussed previously, PtdIns-3-P, PtdIns-3,4-P_2, and PtdIns-3,4,5-P_3 are not substrates for any of the cloned or purified PLCs

(Lips *et al.*, 1989; Serunian *et al.*, 1989). Although a PLC specific for the novel polyphosphoinositides may yet be found, the addition of ^{32}P-labeled lipids to cell lysates does not result in the conversion to inositol phosphates under a variety of conditions (L. A. Serunian, K. R. Auger, and H. Adari, unpublished observations; Lips and Majerus, 1989). In addition, a partially characterized phosphomonoesterase has been reported to be specific for the D-3 phosphate of PtdIns-3-P (Lips and Majerus, 1989). All evidence to date strongly supports the hypothesis that the lipids themselves may be the actual messengers involved in controlling cellular processes.

A number of reports have provided evidence that PtdIns-4-P and PtdIns-4,5-P_2 directly regulate events such as profilactin interactions (Lassing and Lindberg, 1985) and gelsolin function (Janmey and Stossel, 1987) under physiological conditions (Janmey and Stossel, 1989). In addition, these lipids tightly associate with gCap39, another Ca^{2+}- and polyphosphoinositide-regulated protein that effects the polymerization of actin (Yu *et al.*, 1990). Furthermore, a recent report has indicated that profilin can also effect PtdInsP_2 hydrolysis by PLC (Goldschmidt-Clermont *et al.*, 1990). So it appears that not only do the polyphosphoinositides effect the polymerization of actin, but also that a protein important for actin polymerization (profilin) can effect polyphosphoinositide metabolism.

The conventional polyphosphoinositides have also been shown to regulate direct protein–protein interactions that are critical for cell shape (Anderson and Marchesi, 1985). The interaction between glycophorin and protein 4.1 in the red blood cell membrane is important for the integrity of the cell membrane skeleton, and the interaction between these two proteins is mediated by polyphosphoinositides (Anderson and Marchesi, 1985).

Polyphosphoinositides can interact with proteins other than with structural proteins that determine cell shape. Polyphosphoinositides could have important roles in the cell nucleus as regulators of an RNA-dependent ATPase in the nuclear membrane (Smith and Wells, 1984) and as regulators of DNA polymerase α (Sylvia *et al.*, 1988). All of these examples involve the conventional polyphosphoinositides (i.e., PtdIns-4-P and PtdIns-4,5-P_2). It has yet to be determined whether any of the D-3 phosphorylated polyphosphoinositides play similar roles in the regulation of these proteins.

Current evidence supports the idea that the novel polyphosphoinositides are involved in cytoskeletal reorganization. A mutated PDGF receptor (ΔKI), constructed by Severinsson *et al.* (1990) and similar to the construct previously described as being defective in PtdIns 3-kinase association, was unable to induce either actin reorganization or mitogenesis, in contrast to the wild-type transfectant (Severinsson *et al.*, 1990).

Thus, the lack of association of PtdIns 3-kinase correlates with the lack of actin reorganization and the mitogenic signal. Further work is necessary to determine the cellular targets of these novel lipids.

Acknowledgments

We thank Leslie Serunian for helpful discussions concerning the manuscript. Support for much of this work was from National Institutes of Health grants GM 36624 and GM 41890 to L.C.C.

References

Anderson, R. A., and Marchesi, V. T. (1985). *Nature (London)* **318,** 295–298.
Auger, K. R. (1991). Ph.D. thesis. Tufts University School of Medicine, Boston, Massachusetts.
Auger, K. R., Carpenter, C. L., Cantley, L. C., and Varticovski, L. (1989a). *J. Biol. Chem.* **264,** 20181–20184.
Auger, K. R., Serunian, L. A., Soltoff, S. P., Libby, P., and Cantley, L. C. (1989b). *Cell* **57,**167–175.
Berridge, M. J. (1987). *Biochim. Biophys. Acta* **907,** 33–45.
Bjorge, J. D., Chan, T. O., Antczak, M., Kung, H. J., and Fujita, D. J. (1990). *Proc. Natl. Acad. Sci. U.S.A.* **87,** 3816–3820.
Cantley, L. C., Auger, K. R., Carpenter, C., Duckworth, B., Graziani, A., Kapeller, R., and Soltoff, S. (1991). *Cell* **64,** 281–302.
Carmichael, G., Schaffhausen, B. S., Mandel, G., Liang, T. J., and Benjamin, T. L. (1984). *Proc. Natl. Acad. Sci. U.S.A.* **81,** 679–683.
Carpenter, C. L., and Cantley, L. C. (1990). *Biochemistry* **29,** 11147–11156.
Carpenter, C. L., Duckworth, B. C., Auger, K. R., Cohen, B., Schaffhausen, B. S., and Cantley, L. C. (1990). *J. Biol. Chem.* **265,** 19704–19711.
Chan, T. O., Tanaka, A., Bjorge, J. D., and Fujita, D. J. (1990). *Mol. Cell. Biol.* **10,** 3280–3283.
Cohen, B., Yoakim, M., Piwnica-Worms, H., Roberts, T. M., and Schaffhausen, B. S. (1990). *Proc. Natl. Acad. Sci. U.S.A.* **87,** 4458–4462.
Coughlin, S. R., Escobedo, J. A., and Williams, L. T. (1989). *Science* **243,** 1191–1194.
Courtneidge, S. A., and Heber, A. (1987). *Cell* **50,** 1031–1037.
Cunningham, T. W., Lips, D. L., Bansal, V. S., Caldwell, K. K., Mitchell, C. A., and Majerus, P. W. (1990). *J. Biol. Chem.* **265,** 21676–21683.
Diringer, H., and Friis, R. R. (1977). *Cancer Res.* **37,** 2979–2984.
Downes, C. P., Hawkins, P. T., and Irvine, R. F. (1986). *Biochem. J.* **238,** 501–506.
Druker, B. J., Ling, L. E., Cohen, B., Roberts, T. M., and Schaffhausen, B. S. (1990). *J. Virol.* **64,** 4454–4461.
Escobedo, J. A., and Williams, L. T. (1988). *Nature (London)* **335,** 85–87.
Fisher, D. B., and Mueller, G. C. (1968). *Proc. Natl. Acad. Sci. U.S.A.* **60,** 1396–1402.
Fry, M. J., Gebhardt, A., Parker, P. J., and Foulkes, J. G. (1985). *EMBO J.* **4,** 3173–3178.
Fukui, Y., and Hanafusa, H. (1989). *Mol. Cell. Biol.* **9,** 1651–1658.

Fukui, Y., Kornbluth, S., Jong, S.-M., Wang, L.-H., and Hanafusa, H. (1989). *Oncogene Res.* **4,** 283–292.

Goldschmidt-Clermont, P. J., Machesky, L. M., Baldassare, J. J., and Pollard, T. D. (1990). *Science* **247,** 1575–1578.

Graziani, A., Ling, L. E., Endemann, G., Carpenter, C. L., and Cantley, L. C. (1992). *Biochem. J.* (in press).

Graziani, Y., Erikson, E., and Erikson, R. L. (1983). *J. Biol. Chem.* **258,** 2126–2129.

Gutkind, J. S., Lacal, P. M., and Robbins, K. C. (1990). *Mol. Cell. Biol.* **10,** 3806–3809.

Hawkins, P. T., Stephens, L., and Downes, C. P. (1986). *Biochem. J.* **238,** 507–516.

Jackowski, S., Rettenmier, C. W., Sherr, C. J., and Rock, C. O. (1986). *J. Biol. Chem.* **261,** 4978–4985.

Janmey, P. A., and Stossel, T. P. (1987). *Nature (London)* **325,** 362–364.

Janmey, P. A., and Stossel, T. P. (1989). *J. Biol. Chem.* **264,** 4825–4831.

Kaplan, D. R., Whitman, M., Schaffhausen, B., Raptis, L., Garcea, R. L., Pallas, D., Roberts, T. M., and Cantley, L. (1986). *Proc. Natl. Acad. Sci. U.S.A.* **83,** 3624–3628.

Kaplan, D. R., Whitman, M., Schaffhausen, B., Pallas, D. C., White, M., Cantley, L., and Roberts, T. M. (1987). *Cell* **50,** 1021–1029.

Kazlauskas, A., and Cooper, J. A. (1989). *Cell* **58,** 1121–1133.

Kazlauskas, A., and Cooper, J. A. (1990). *EMBO J.* **9,** 3279–3286.

Kucera, G. L., and Rittenhouse, S. E. (1990). *J. Biol. Chem.* **265,** 5345–5348.

Lassing, I., and Lindberg, U. (1985). *Nature (London)* **314,** 472–474.

Lips, D. L., and Majerus, P. W. (1989). *J. Biol. Chem.* **264,** 19911–19915.

Lips, D. L., Majerus, P. W., Gorga, F. R., Young, A. T., and Benjamin, T. L. (1989). *J. Biol. Chem.* **264,** 8759–8763.

Macara, I. G., Marinetti, G. V., and Balduzzi, P. C. (1984). *Proc. Natl. Acad. Sci. U.S.A.* **81,** 2728–2732.

Nolan, R. D., and Lapetina, E. G. (1990). *J. Biol. Chem.* **265,** 2441–2445.

Nolan, R. D., and Lapetina, E. G. (1991). *Biochem. Biophys. Res. Commun.* **174,** 524–528.

Oostra, B. A., Harvey, R., Ely, B. K., Markham, A. F., and Smith, A. E. (1983). *Nature (London)* **304,** 456–459.

Pignataro, O. P., and Ascoli, M. (1990). *J. Biol. Chem.* **265,** 1718–1723.

Piwnica-Worms, H., Kaplan, D. R., Whitman, M., and Roberts, T. M. (1986). *Mol. Cell. Biol.* **6,** 2033–2040.

Piwnica-Worms, H., Williams, N. G., Cheng, S. H., and Roberts, T. M. (1990). *J. Virol.* **64,** 61–68.

Rana, R. S., and Hokin, L. E. (1990). *Physiol. Rev.* **70,** 115–164.

Richert, N. D., Blithe, D. L., and Pastan, I. (1982). *J. Biol. Chem.* **257,** 7143–7150.

Roussel, M. F., Shurtleff, S. A., Downing, J. R., and Sherr, C. J. (1990). *Proc. Natl. Acad. Sci. U.S.A.* **87,** 6738–6742.

Ruderman, N. B., Kapeller, R., White, M. F., and Cantley, L. C. (1990). *Proc. Natl. Acad.Sci. U.S.A.* **87,** 1411–1415.

Santiago-Calvo, E., Mule, S. J., and Hokin, L. W. (1963). *Biochim. Biophys. Acta* **70,** 91–93.

Santiago-Calvo, E., Mule, C. M., Hokin, M. R., and Hokin, L. W. (1964). *Biochim. Biophys. Acta* **84,** 550–562.

Serunian, L. A., Haber, M. T., Fukui, T., Kim, J. W., Rhee, S. G., Lowenstein, J. M., and Cantley, L. C. (1989). *J. Biol. Chem.* **264,** 17809–17815.

Serunian, L. A., Auger, K. R., Roberts, T., and Cantley, L. C. (1990). *J. Virol.* **64,** 4718–4725.

Severinsson, L., Ek, B., Mellstrom, K., Claesson-Welsh, L., and Heldin, C.-H. (1990). *Mol. Cell. Biol.* **10,** 801–809.

Smith, C. D., and Wells, W. W. (1984). *J. Biol. Chem.* **259,** 11890–11894.

Stephens, L., Hawkins, P. T., and Downes, C. P. (1989). *Biochem. J.* **259,** 267–276.
Sugimoto, Y., Whitman, M., Cantley, L. C., and Erikson, R. L. (1984). *Proc. Natl. Acad. Sci. U.S.A.* **81,** 2117–2121.
Sylvia, V., Curtin, G., Norman, J., Stec, J., and Busbee, D. (1988). *Cell* **54,** 651–658.
Talmage, D. A., Freund, R., Young, A. T., Dahl, J., Dawe, C. J., and Benjamin, T. L. (1989). *Cell* **59,** 55–65.
Traynor-Kaplan, A. E., Harris, A. L., Thompson, B. L., Taylor, P., and Sklar, L. A. (1988). *Nature (London)* **334,** 353–356.
Traynor-Kaplan, A. E., Thompson, B. L., Harris, A. L., Taylor, P., Omann, G. M., and Sklar, L. A. (1989). *J. Biol. Chem.* **264,** 15668–15673.
Ulug, E. T., Hawkins, P. T., Hanley, M. R., and Courtneidge, S. A. (1990). *J. Virol.* **64,** 3895–3904.
Vadnal, R. E., and Parthasarathy, R. (1989). *Biochem. Biophys. Res. Commun.* **163,** 995–1001.
Varticovski, L., Drucker, B., Morrison, D., Cantley, L., and Roberts, T. (1989). *Nature (London)* **342,** 699–702.
Weinstein, I. B. (1987). *J. Cell. Biochem.* **33,** 213–244.
Whitman, M., and Cantley, L. (1988). *Biochim. Biophys. Acta* **948,** 327–344.
Whitman, M., Kaplan, D. R., Schaffhausen, B., Cantley, L., and Roberts, T. M. (1985). *Nature (London)* **315,** 239–242.
Whitman, M., Kaplan, D., Roberts, T., and Cantley, L. (1987). *Biochem. J.* **247,** 165–174.
Whitman, M., Downes, C. P., Keeler, M., Keller, T., and Cantley, L. (1988). *Nature (London)* **332,** 644–646.
Williams, L. T. (1989). *Science* **243,** 1564–1570.
Yamamoto, K., Graziani, A., Carpenter, C. L., Cantley, L. C., and Lapetina, E. G. (1990). *J. Biol. Chem.* **265,** 22086–22089.
Yu, F.-X., Johnston, P. A., Sudhof, T. C., and Yin, H. L. (1990). *Science* **250,** 1413–1415.

Index